A PRACTICAL ENGLISH—CHINESE LIBRARY OF TRADITIONAL CHINESE MEDICINE

PUBLISHING HOUSE OF SHANGHAI UNIVERSITY OF TRADITIONAL CHINESE MEDICINE

EDITOR IN—CHIEF ZHANG ENQIN

BASIC THEORY OF TRADITIONAL CHINESE MEDICINE

(I)

Written by Zhang Enqin
Translated by Zhang Enqin

Revised by Xu Guoqian

Translated by Xu Xiangcai

Revised by Wang Zhikui

英汉对照
实用中医文库

主　编　张恩勤

中医基础理论

●上册

编译　张恩勤
审校　徐国仟
翻译　徐象才
审校　王治奎

上海中医药大学出版社

THE EDITING AND TRANSLATING COMMITTEE OF THE LIBRARY

《英汉对照实用中医文库》编译委员会

Specially Invited International Editors

特邀外籍审校人员

Preface

The books in series, entitled "*A Practical English-Chinese Library of Traditional Chinese Medicine*", are edited with a view to disseminating the theory and knowledge of traditional Chinese medicine (TCM) across the world, promoting academic exchanges on medical science between China and other countries, and meeting with the ever-increasing international interest in TCM, so as to make it serve the interests of all nations and benefit entire mankind. This library is the first of its kind in China.

The library is composed of 12 books: ***Basic Theory of TCM*** (in two volumes), ***Diagnostics of TCM, The Chinese Materia Medica, Prescriptions of TCM, Clinic of TCM*** (in two volumes), ***Health Preservation and Rehabilitation, Chinese Acupuncture and Moxibustion, Chinese Medicated Diet*** and ***Chinese Qigong***. The two other English-Chinese books —— ***Rare Chinese Materia Medica*** and ***Highly Efficacious Chinese Patent Medicine*** —— chiefly edited by me are also published simultaneously along with this library.

The authors and editors of the series strive to abide by the following principles: maintaining the systematism, integrity, practicability and adaptability in terms of TCM theory; paying full attention to the organic connection between basic theory and clinical treatment, taking in the available results of scientific researches carried out at home and abroad in the field of TCM; and being concise, precise, and easy to undeistand in the Chinese version, and correct and fluent in the English one. Some of the books mentioned above contain figures and coloured photos. It is our sincere hope that the books will turn out to be good teachers and reliable friends of those abroad who have begun to learn and practise TCM and Chinese, and provide help for those at home who wish to study TCM documents in English.

The component books of this library are written, translated, and edited through joint efforts of professors, associate professors, lecturers and medical research workers from Shandong TCM College and its affiliated hospital, Shandong Medical University and its affiliated hospital, Shandong University, Shandong Teachers Training University, Shandong Medical Academy, Shandong Provincial Anti-epidemic Station, China Academy of TCM, Nanjing TCM College, Shanghai TCM College, Beijing TCM College, etc.

In order to ensure that the present library is of good quality, we have sent its Chinese version for revision to Professor Zhou Fengwu, Professor Li Keshao who was once my tutor when I was a postgraduate student, Professor Xu Guoqian and Professor Zhang Zhenyu at Shandong TCM College, Professor Qiu Maoliang at Nanjing TCM College, and Professor Lu Tongjie, director of the Affiliated Hospital of Shandong TCM College; and the English version for proofreading to Professor Huang Xiaokai of Beijiug Medical University, Professor Lu Chengzhi, head of the Foreign Languages Department of Shandong Medical University, Professoı Huang Jiade of Shandong Univeısity, Mr. Huang Wenxing, professor of pharmacology, Mme. Zou Ling, professor of gynecology and obstetrics, both working in Shandong Medical University, and our foreign friends, Ms. Beth Hocks, Australian teacher of English, Mr. Howard G. Adams, American teacher of English, and some others working in Jinan.

I am deeply indebted to Mr. Li Dichen, Editor-in-Chief of Publishing House of Shanghai TCM College, and his colleagues, Mme. Xu Ping, director of the Editorial Depatmrent, and Mr. Yao Yong, responsible editor, for their advice about drawing up an outline for compiling the library to ensure a success of it; to Mr. Chen Keji, professor of China Academy of TCM and advisor on traditional medicine to WHO, Professor Zhang Zhiyuan and Associate Professor Shao Guanyong of Shandong TCM College, Mr. Liu Chonggang, deputy head of the Yellow River Publishing House, for their valuable, instructive suggestions; and to responsible members at various levels, such as Mr. Hu Ximing, Chairman of the World Acupuncture and Moxibustion Association, vice-minister of the Ministry of public Health and chief of the Administrative Bureau of TCM and Pharmacy of the People's Republic of China, Mr. Zou Jilong, president of Shandong TCM College, Mr. Yan Shiyun, vice-president of Shanghai TCM College, Mr. Gao Heting, president of Beijing TCM College, Mr. Xiang Ping, vice president of Nanjing TCM College, and Mr. Shang Zhichang, president of Henan TCM College for their warm encouragement and indispensable support as well as their personal participation in compiling and checking the books.

TCM, which dates back to ancient times, has a unique

and profound theoretical system. The greater part of its terminology has particular denotations, and is matter-of-factly difficult to understand and translate. Inaccuracies in the library, therefore, are unavoidable. I hope that my friends in the TCM circle will oblige me with timely corrections.

May TCM spread all over the world and everyone under the heaven enjoy a long happy life.

May 20th, 1988 Dr. Zhang Enqin

Editor-in-Chief of ***A Practical English-Chinese Library of Traditional Chinese Medicine,*** Director of the Advanced Studies Department of Shandong TCM College

前　言

为扩大中医学在国际上的影响，促进中外医学学术交流，适应国外日趋发展的“中医热”形势，使传统的中医学走向世界，造福人类，我们编写了这套《英汉对照实用中医文库》。在国内，这尚属首部。

该文库包括《中医基础理论》(上、下册)、《中医诊断学》、《中药学》、《方剂学》、《中医临床各科》(上、下册)、《中医养生康复学》、《中国针灸》、《中国推拿》、《中国药膳》和《中国气功》，共十二个分册。与《文库》同时出版的还有其配套书——英汉对照《中国名贵药材》和《中国名优中成药》。

《英汉对照实用中医文库》的编译宗旨是：在理论上，努力保持中医学体系的系统性、完整性，突出实用性和针对性；在内容上，充分注意基础理论与临床治疗的有机联系，汲取国内外已公布的科研成果，以反映当代中医学术水平；在文字上，力求中文简明扼要，通俗易懂，译文准确流畅，并配有图表、彩照。我们竭诚希望《英汉对照实用中医文库》能成为国外读者学习中医、汉语的良师益友，同时也为国内读者学习中医专业英语提供帮助。

负责文库编写、翻译和审校的主要是山东中医学院及其附属医院、山东医科大学及其附属医院、山东大学、山东师范大学、山东省医学科学院、山东省卫生防疫站、中国中医研究院、南京中医学院，上海中医学院和北京中医学院等单位的部分教授、副教授、讲师和科研人员。

为确保文库质量，各分册中文稿还先后承蒙山东中医学院周凤梧教授、李克绍教授、徐国仟教授、张珍玉教授，南京中医学院邱茂良教授，山东中医学院附属医院院长吕同杰教授等审阅；英文稿先后承蒙北京医科大学英语教研室黄孝楷教授，山东医科大学英语教研室主任卢承志教授，山东大学外文系黄嘉德教授，山东医科大学药理教研室黄文兴教授、妇产科教研室邹玲教授以及澳大利亚籍教师 Beth Hocks 女士和美籍教师 Howard G. Adams 先生等审阅。

上海中医学院出版社总编辑李迪臣、编辑部主任徐平和责任编辑姚勇，亲自帮助我们修订编写大纲，指导编译工作；世界卫生组织传统医学顾问、中国中医研究院陈可冀教授，山东中医学院张志远教授、邵冠勇副教授，黄河出版社副社长刘崇刚，也为本文库的编译工作提出了许多宝贵的指导性意见；编译工作还得到了各级领导的支持和帮助，世界针灸学会联合会主席、中华人民共和国卫生部副部长兼国家中医药管理局局长胡熙明先生，山东中医学院院长邹积隆先生，上海中医学院副院长严世芸先生，北京中医学院院长高鹤亭先生，南京中医学院副院长项平先生和河南中医学院院长尚炽昌先生等，亲自参加编审并给予指导，在此一并表示衷心感谢！

由于中医学源远流长，其理论体系独特，不少名词术语深奥难解，译成英文，难度较大。故书中错误、欠妥之处在所难免，敬希国内外同道指正。

愿中医流传世界，求普天下人健康长寿。

主编　张恩勤

1988年5月20日

CONTENTS

目　录

Basic Theory of Traditional Chinese Medicine (I)

中医基础理论（上册）

Chapter One

Introduction

Section 1

Beginning, Growth and Present State of Traditional Chinese Medicine

Traditional Chinese Medicine (TCM) has a long history. In remote antiquity, our ancestors created primitive medicine during their struggles against nature. While searching for food they found that some foods had the specific property of relieving or eliminating certain diseases. That was the beginning of finding and using herbal medicines. While warming themselves around a fire they discovered that the way of local warming with hot stones or earth wrapped in bark or animal skin would relieve or eliminate certain symptoms of diseases. They practised and improved this method repeatedly and then gradually brought into being the therapies of hot medicated compress and moxibustion. In the course of using stone implements as tools of production, they noted, by chance, that the pain in one part of the body would be alleviated when some other part was pricked. Then treatment with *bian shi* (stone needles) and bone needles came into being. This gradually resulted in acupuncture therapy. Afterwards the therapy of channels was born.

The theories of TCM come mainly from practice and have been continually enriched and expanded through practice. More than 2,000 years ago ***Canon of Medicine***, the earliest of the extant medical classics in China was produced.

第一章

导论

第一节　中医学的形成、发展与现状

中医有着悠久的历史。早在远古时代，我们的祖先在与大自然作斗争中就创造了原始医学。人们在寻找食物的过程中，发现某些食物能减轻或消除某些病症，这就是发现和应用中药的起源；在烘火取暖的基础上，发现用兽皮、树皮包上烧热的石块或沙土作局部取暖可消除某些病痛，通过反复实践和改进，逐渐产生了热熨法和灸法；在使用石器作为生产工具的过程中，发现人体某一部位受到刺伤后反能解除另一部位的病痛，从而创造了运用砭石、骨针治病的方法，并在此基础上，逐渐发展为针刺疗法，进而形成了经络学说。

中医理论主要来源于实践，并在实践中不断得到充实和发展。早在两千多年前，中国现存最早的中医理论专著《黄帝内经》（即

It was known to later generations as two books: ***Plain Questions*** and ***Miraculous Pivot***. The latter is also called ***Canon of Acupuncture*** or ***Nine Volumes***. The book, ***Canon of Medicine***, extensively summarizes and systematizes the previous experiences of treatment and theories of medicine, deals at length with the anatomy, physiology and pathology of the human body, and the diagnosis, treatment and prevention of diseases, on the basis of the then achievements of other natural sciences, and under the guidance of the ancient naive materialism and spontaneous dialectics. It lays a primary foundation for the theories of TCM. ***Classic on Medical Problems*** is a classical medical treatise which can match ***Canon of Medicine***. It was published before the Han dynasty (206B.C.—220A.D.). Legend has it that the book was compiled by Qin Yueren. It also deals with physiology, pathology, diagnosis, treatment and so on, replenishing what ***Canon of Medicine*** lacks.

From the Qin and Han dynasties (221 B.C.—220A.D.), doctors in the interior of China began to prescribe more and more rhinoceros horn (*Cornu Rhinocerotis*), amber (*Succinum*), antelope's horn (*Cornu Antelopis*) and musk (*Moschus*) from the minority nationalities; longan pulp (*Arillus Longan*), lychee-seed (*Semen Litchi*) from the South China Sea and even medical materials from Southeast Asia and other regions as a result of ever-developing communications and transportation both inside and outside of China. This enriched the Chinese people's knowledge of medicine. The book ***The Herbal*** is the earliest extant classic on materia medica handed down from that time. It is the summary of pharmaceutical knowledge which was known before the Han dynasty. Not only does it discuss in great detail 365 kinds of drugs but also records and narrates the pharmacological theories of "*Jun, Chen, Zuo and Shi*" (monarch, minister, assistant and guide) indicating the different actions of drugs in a prescription, "*Qi Qing He*

后世之《素问》和《灵枢》两书，后者亦称《针经》、《九卷》）问世。该书系统总结了在此之前的治疗经验和医学理论，结合当时的其他自然科学成就，运用朴素的唯物论和自发的辨证法思想，对人体的解剖、生理、病理以及疾病的诊断、治疗与预防，做了比较全面的阐述，初步奠定了中医学的理论基础。《难经》是一部与《黄帝内经》相媲美的古典医籍，成书于汉之前，相传系秦越人所著。其内容亦包括生理、病理、诊断、治疗等各个方面，补充了《黄帝内经》之不足。

秦汉以来，内外交通日渐发达，少数民族地区的犀角、琥珀、羚羊角、麝香，以及南海的龙眼、荔枝核等，渐为内地医家所采用。东南亚等地的药材也不断进入中国，从而丰富了人们的药材知识。《神农本草经》就是当时流传下来的、中国现存最早的药物学专著。它总结了汉以前人们的药物知识，载药365种，并记述

He" (seven conditions in making up prescriptions) "*Si Qi*" (four properties of drugs,) "*Wu Wei*" (five kinds of flavours: sour, bitter, sweet, acrid and salty) and so on. Long-term clinical practice and modern scientific researches have proved that most of the effects of the drugs recorded in this book are true, as with Chinese ephedra (*Herba Ephedrae*) used in the treatment of asthma, goldthread root (*Rhizoma Coptidis*) prescribed in dysentery, kelp (*Sargassum*) prescribed in goiter and so on.

Zhang Zhongjing, a famous TCM doctor in the Eastern Han dynasty (300 A.D.), made thorough study of such classics as ***Plain Questions, Canon of Acupuncture, Classic on Medical Problems*** and the like. Meanwhile he collected extensively other effective prescriptions. At last he wrote a book by combining what he had learned with his own findings in clinical practice. The book's title is ***Treatise on Febrile Diseases and Miscellaneous Diseases.*** It analyses and differentiates febrile diseases according to the theory of six channels, miscellaneous diseases according to the pathological changes of viscera and bowels and their interrelations, and in so doing establishes Chinese medicine's theoretical system and therapeutic principle, i.e., diagnosis and treatment based on an overall analysis of signs and symptoms. It lays a foundation for the development of clinical medicine. Later generations divided it into two books. One is ***Treatise on Febrile Diseases*** in which there are 113 prescriptions (among them is one named "*Yu Yu Liang* Pill" which exists only in name). The other is ***Synopsis of Prescriptions of Golden Chamber.*** It introduces 262 prescriptions, some of which are the same as those stated in the former book. Hence, the number of the prescriptions from these two books is up to 269 in all. They contain, basically, the prescriptions often used in every department of clinical medicine and are known as the earliest ancestor of all the other books on the study of prescriptions.

了君、臣、佐、使、七情和合、四气五味等药物学理论。长期临床实践和现代科学研究证明：该书所载药效大多是正确的，如麻黄治喘，黄连治痢，海藻治瘿等。

公元三世纪，东汉著名医家张仲景在深入钻研《素问》、《针经》、《难经》等古典医籍的基础上，广泛采集众人的有效药方，并结合自己的临床经验，著成《伤寒杂病论》。该书以六经辨伤寒，以脏腑辨杂病，确立了中医学辨证施治的理论体系与治疗原则，为临床医学的发展奠定了基础。后世又将该书分为《伤寒论》和《金匮要略》。其中，《伤寒论》载方113首(实为112首，因其中的禹余粮丸有方无药)，《金匮要略》载方262首，除去重复，两书实收方剂269首，基本上概括了临床各科的常用方剂，被誉为“方书之祖”。

Huang Fumi (215—282 A.D.), a noted medical man in the Western Jin dynasty, compiled the book, ***A-B Classic of Acupuncture and Moxibustion*** by rearranging the basic contents of the three books: ***Plain Questions, Canon of Acupuncture*** and ***An Outline of Points for Acupuncture and Moxibustion.*** The book, ***A-B Classic of Acupuncture and Moxibustion,*** consists of 12 volumes, 128 chapters and is the earliest extant classic on acupuncture and moxibustion in China. Not only does it refer to viscera and bowels, channels and collaterals, acupuncture points, pathogenesis, diagnosis, acupuncture manipulation, puncture contraindication, indication of acupuncture points and so on, but also verifies the total number of the acupoints of that time and gives a list of 349 point locations (49 individual points and 300 double points). What is more, it also discusses the therapeutic properties of each point in each part of the body and its prohibitions, and summarizes the methods of manipulaton of needles. It has exerted a great influence upon the medicine of acupuncture and moxibustion all over the world. It was stipulated by the Japanese authorities as early as 701 A.D. as one of the required reading books for B.M. candidates.

In 610 A.D. ,Chao Yuanfang, together with others, compiled the book ***General Treatise on the Causes and Symptoms of Diseases*** which is the earliest extant classic on etiology and syndrome in China. It is of 50 volumes, divided into 67 categories, and lists 1,700 syndromes and expounds respectively the pathology, signs and symptoms of various diseases concerning internal medicine, surgery, gynaecology, pediatrics as well as the five sense organs. The book contains detailed and precise descriptions of the etiology and pathogenesis of certain diseases. For instance, it points out clearly that some parasitic infections have a lot to do with diet, and holds that taeniasis results from eating raw meat. In addition, it records many operations such as intestinal anastomosis, artificial abor-

西晋医家皇甫谧(公元215～282)将《素问》、《针经》、《明堂孔穴针灸治要》三书的基本内容，进行重新归类编排，撰成《针灸甲乙经》12卷，128篇。该书为中国现存最早的一部针灸专书，其内容包括脏腑、经络、腧穴、病机、诊断、针刺手法、刺禁腧穴主治等。书中经过考查确定了当时的腧穴总数和穴位349个(包括单穴49个，双穴300个)，论述了各部穴位的适应证与禁忌，总结了操作手法等，对世界针灸医学影响很大。公元701年日本政府制定医药职令时规定，本书为医学士必修书。

公元610年，巢元方等人集体编写的《诸病源候论》，是中国现存最早的病因证候学专著。全书共50卷，分67门，载列证候1,700余条，分别论述了内、外、妇、儿、五官等各种疾病的病因病理和症状。其中对一些疾病的病因及发病原理已描述得比较详尽而科学。例如：对某些寄生虫的感染，已明确指出与饮食有关；认为绦虫病系吃不熟的肉类所致。书中还记载了肠吻合术、

tion, tooth extraction. This shows that surgery reached rather a high level at that time.

In the time of the Sui and Tang dynasties, China was politically unified, became prosperous in economy and culture and enjoyed rapid development in internal and external communication and transportation, both resulting in the import of more and more medicinal materials and in the ever enriching of the experience of physicians in administering drugs. Then came the time when the achievements in pharmacology needed to be further summarized. In 657 A.D., the government of the Tang dynasty instructed Su Jing to head about 20 physicians in correcting and recompiling the book, ***Chinese Materia Medica***. This job was finished in 659 A.D., and a new book entitled ***The Newly-revised Materia Medica in the Tang Dynasty*** or ***The Tang Materia Medica***. It is the first pharmacopoeia of its kind enforced by the government in ancient China, and the earliest state-promulgated pharmacopoeia in the world. It is 883 years older than the "Nuremberg Pharmacopoeia" enforced by the government of Nuremberg in Europe in 1542 A.D.. This pharmacopoeia has 54 volumes altogether, comprising three parts: materia medica, drug illustrations, and statements of illustrations. It deals with 850 drugs and has exerted a great influence outside China In 713 A.D., the Japanese government stipulated that its private copies which were being circulated among the common people, should be used as an obligatory textbook for medical students.

Sun Simiao (581—682 A.D.), a famous medical man in the Tang dynasty, devoted his life to writing out the two books: ***Prescriptions Worth a Thousand Gold for Emergencies*** and ***A Supplement to the Essential Prescriptions Worth a Thousand Gold***. The former is divided into 30 volumes and introduces 5,300 prescriptions; the latter, 30 volumes, 2,571 prescriptions. These two books deal with the key problems

人工流产、拔牙等手术，说明当时的外科手术已达到较高的水平。

隋唐时期，由于政治统一，经济文化繁荣，内外交通发达，外来药物日益增多，用药经验不断丰富，对药物学成就进一步总结已成为当时的客观需要。公元657年唐政府组织苏敬等二十余人集体编修本草，于公元659年完稿，名为《唐·新修本草》（又名《唐本草》）。这是中国古代由政府颁行的第一部药典，也是世界上最早的国家药典。它比欧州纽伦堡政府公元1542年颁行的《纽伦堡药典》早883年。该书共54卷，包括本草、药图、图经三部分，载药850种，在国外影响较大。公元713年，日本官方就以此书的传抄本规定为学医的必读课本。

唐代医家孙思邈（公元581～682）集毕生之精力，著成《备急千金要方》、《千金翼方》。其中，《千金要方》分为30卷，合方论5,300首；《千金翼方》亦30卷，载方2,571首。二书还对临床

of every clinical department: acupuncture and moxibustion, diet therapy, prevention, health preservation and so on. His outstanding achievement is in the treatment of deficiency diseases. For example, he realized that patients suffering from goiter and the like were among those who lived in the mountains for a long time and drank a type of harmful water. He dissuaded people from living for any length of time in such places and advocated that nyctalopes should be treated with animals' livers, to mention but a few. In 752 A.D., Wang Tao wrote a treatise, ***The Medical Secrets of An Official.*** The book contains 40 volumes, 1,104 categories (of which 1,048 have so far been verified) and introduces 6,000 or so prescriptions. It can certainly be known as a mastery of prescriptions available before the Tang dynasty.

In the Song dynasty (960—1279 A.D.), more attention was paid to education in terms of TCM. The government set up the Imperial Medical Bureau, which was then the highest organ for cultivating qualified Chinese medical men. The courses designated for the students were ***Plain Qestions Classic on Medical Problems***, ***Treatise on Febrile Diseases***, ***General Treatise on the Causes and Symptoms of Diseases*** and so on. Also, the teaching methods were improved greatly. For example, in 1026 A.D., Wang Weiyi, a specialist in acupuncture and moxibustion, designed two life-size [bronze figures and had them cast for use in teaching and examining the personnel learning acupuncture and moxibustion. Both o. them have the 12 channels and the exact locations ot 354 points marked by carving or piercing caretully on their surfaces. When used tor the purpose of testing, they were filled with water and coated with beeswax by the examiner ahead of time. It a candidate spotted and punctured the right point, water would issue from it. That was, indeed, a creative effort in the educational cause of Chinese medicine. In 1057 A.D., in the Song dynasty, a special organ called "Bureau for Cor-

各科、针灸、食疗、预防、养生等均有论述。尤其在营养缺乏性疾病防治方面，成就突出。如他认为瘿病(指甲状腺肿类疾病)是因人们久居山区，长期饮用一种不好的水所致，劝告人们不要久居这些地方；对夜盲病人，采用动物肝脏治疗等。公元752年，王焘著成《外台秘要》，全书共40卷，1,104门(据今核实为1,048门)，载方6,000余首，可谓集唐以前方书之大成。

宋代对中医教育比较重视。宋政府设立“太医局”，作为培养中医人材的最高机构。学生所学课程包括《素问》、《难经》、《伤寒论》和《诸病源候论》等。教学方法也有很大改进，如针灸医官王惟一曾设计铸造铜人两具(公元1026年)，精细刻制了十二经脉和354个穴位，作为针灸教学和考试医师之用。考试时，试官将铜人穴位注水，外用蜡封。受试者如取穴正确，可针进水出。这是中国医学教育事业的创举。公元1057年，宋政府专设“校正

recting Medical Books" was set up in order to collect, sort out, research textually and collate the medical books ot past ages. Ten years later, in about 1068—1077 A.D., a number of collated book were printed and published in succession. Among others now available are ***Plain Questions, Treatise on Febrile Diseases, Synopsis of Prescriptions of the Golden Chamber, A-B Classic of Acupuncture and Moxibustion, General Treatise on the Causes and Symptoms of Diseases, Prescriptions Worth a Thousand Gold for Emergencies, A Supplement to The Essential Prescriptions Worth a Thousand Gold, The Medical Secrets of An Official*** and so on, which have been handed down after being checked and printed.

In the times of the Jin and Yuan dynasties (1200—1400 A.D.), there appeared many medical schools in the circle ot Chinese medicine, each ot which had its own special features. Four of them are more typical ones. The first one was the School ot Cold and Cool, founded by Liu Wansu (1120—1200 A.D.), who thought that the various signs and symptoms ot the disease, "*shang han*", (which is a general term for febrile diseases due to exogenous pathogenic factors) foten had something to do with fire and heat evils, so drugs of a cold and cool nature should be used in treating it. The second was the School of Attacking or Purgating headed by Zhang Congzheng (1156—1228 A.D.), who held that disease resulted from the invasion of exopathic factors into the human body, that as soon as a disease was found, efforts should be made to dispel the exopathic factors, and that three methods often served this purpose, namely, diaphoresis, emesis and purgation. The third school was represented by Li Dongyuan (1180—1251 A.D.), who believed that "The internal injuries of the spleen and stomach were the cause of many kinds of diseases.", so the most important thing in treatment should be to warm and invigorate the spleen and stomach." Because the spleen was included in the "earth" so far as the theory of five elem-

医书局”，有计划地对历代重要医籍进行了搜集、整理、考证和校勘，历时十余年，约在1068～1077年陆续刊行。目前我们所能读到的《素问》、《伤寒论》、《金匮要略》、《针灸甲乙经》、《诸病源候论》、《千金要方》、《千金翼方》和《外台秘要》等，都是经过此次校订、刊行后流传下来的。

公元十二至十四世纪的金元时代，中医学出现了许多各具特色的医学流派。其中有代表性的有四大家、即：刘完素（公元1120～1200），认为伤寒（泛指发热性疾病）的各种症状多与“火热”有关，因而在治疗上多用寒凉药物，被后世称之为“寒凉派”；张从正（约公元1156～1228），认为病由外邪侵入人体所生，一经致病，就应祛邪，故治疗多用汗、吐、下三法以攻邪，被后世称之为“攻下派”；李东垣（公元1180～1251），提出“内伤脾胃，百病由生”，治疗时重在温补脾胃，因脾在五行学说中属“土”，故被后世称之

ents is concerned, this school was known as the School of Nourishing the Earth. The fourth one was the School of Nourishing the Essence. Its founder was Zhu Zhenheng (1281—1358 A.D.). He thought that *yang* (the functional aspect of internal organs) was usually in excess while *yin* (the structural aspect of internal organs) was ever deficient, i.e., the *yang* of the body was often excessive, while the *yin* was deficient; so nourishing the essence and purging the fire should be the chief measures taken in treating diseases.

Li Shizhen (1518—1593 A.D.) was a great physician and pharmacologist in the Ming dynasty. He got a clear understanding of the growing forms of many medicinal plants by going up mountains to pick up medicinal herbs on his own and doing investigations conscientiously in many places, dissecting some medicinal ingredients from animals and watching out for their effects by following their traces, and comparing and refining some medicinal minerals. Meanwhile he consulted more than 800 sorts of documents. In so doing he was able to write his book: ***Compendium of Materia Medica.*** It took him 27 years to accomplish this. The book lists 1,892 medicines and more than 10,000 prescriptions. It is a great contribution to the development of pharmacology both in China and throughout the world.

In about the 11th century A.D., Chinese medicine began to use the variolation method to prevent smallpox, thus becoming the pioneer of immunology in the world. From the 17th to 19th century A.D., infectious diseases spread continually. The School of Epidemic Febrile Diseases appeared and grew in the struggle against them. Wu Youxing, a medical man of this school in the Ming dynasty, thought that the onset of an infectious disease was not due to wind or cold, or summer-heat or dampness, but due to impure, noxious atmospheric influences, which he called foul and evil-foreboding air (epidemic noxious factor). He pointed out that this foul and evil-foreboding

为“补土派”，朱震亨(公元1281～1358)，认为人体“阳常有余，阴常不足”(即认为人体常常阳气过盛，阴气不足)，治疗疾病应以养阴降火为主，被后世称之为“养阴派”。

明代医药学家李时珍(公元1518～1593)亲自上山采药，广泛地到各地调查，搞清了许多药用植物的生长形态，并对某些动物药进行解剖或追踪观察，对药用矿物进行比较和炼制，参考文献800余种，历时27年之久，写成了《本草纲目》，收载药物1,892种，附方10,000多个，对中国和世界药物学的发展做出了杰出的贡献。

大约在公元十一世纪，中医即开始应用“人痘接种法”预防天花，成为世界医学免疫学的先驱。公元十七至十九世纪，由于传染病的不断流行，人们在同传染病作斗争的过程中，形成并发展了温病学派。如明代吴有性认为传染病的发生，“非风非寒，非暑非湿，乃天地间别有一种异气所感，”他称之为“戾气”。他指出“戾

air got into the human body by way of the mouth and nose. People, old or young, strong or weak, would fall ill whenever they had the air inside, which marked a breakthrough in the traditional theory of TCM which held that diseases got into the body only through its surface. This is no doubt a great discovery because it occurred in the middle of the 17th century A.D. when bacteriology had not yet been discovered. Up to the Qing dynasty, rich experiences in treating epidemic febrile diseases, including infectious and noninfectious, had been vastly accumulated in TCM. The treatment theory in this respect was further developed, and a new theory concerning the treatment of epidemic febrile diseases was formed, i.e., when treating an epidemic disease one should either analyse, differentiate or judge its development by studying the four conditions or stages of its process — *wei* (superficial defensive) system, *qi* (inner defensive) system, *ying* (constructive or nutrient) system and *xue* (blood) system or analyse and differentiate it according to the pathological changes of the triple warmer (three phases of febrile diseases: upper, middle and lower). The representative works expounding the above theory are ***Treatise on Epidemic Febrile Diseases*** by Ye Gui, ***Detailed Analysis of Febrile Diseases due to Dampness and Heat*** by Xue Xue, ***Treatise on Differentiation and Treatment of Epidemic Febrile Diseases*** By Wu Tang, (***Compendium on Epidemic Febrile Diseases*** by Wang Shixiong, to mention but a few.

Wang Qingren (1768—1831 A.D.), a medical man in the Qing dynasty, wrote a book entitled ***Corrections on the Errors of Medical Works*** on the basis of what he had discovered during autopsies and his own clinical practice. In his book, he corrected the errors in autopsy in ancient medical books, emphasized the importance of autopsy to a doctor, and developed the theory that blood stasis (including stagnated blood and extravasated blood) would result in diseases, and the methods of treating these kinds of diseases.

气”的传染途径是自口鼻而入，无论表少强弱，触之皆 病。这就突破事中医学历来认为的病邪是由体表进入人体的传统理论，在细菌学尚未出现的十七世纪中叶，这无疑是一伟大创举。到了清代，中医在治疗温病(包括传染性和非传染性发热性疾病)方面积累了大量经验，因而在理论上也有了新的发展，产生了以“卫气营血”和“三焦”对温病进行辨证施治的温热病学说。反映这方面成就的代表著作有叶桂的《温热论》、薛雪的《湿热 条 辨》、吴瑭 的《温病条辨》及王士雄的《温热经纬》等。

清代医家王清任(1768～1831)根据尸体解剖和临床经验写成《医林改错》，改正了古代医书在人体解剖方面的的一些错误，强调了解剖知识对医生的重要性，并发展了瘀血致病理论与治疗方法。

In the last 100 years, with the widespread use of Western medcine in China, a new situation has arisen in which TCM and Western medicine are developing side by side. Many medical workers have come to realize that Chinese medicine and Western medicine have their own advantages. Efforts have been made to combine these two schools and to put forward a series of ideas on how to assimilate the two schools in theory and practice. A new trend or school of combining Chinese and Western medicine has gradually taken shape. Its representative figures and works are as follows: Tang Zonghai (1862—1918 A.D.) and his ***The Five Kinds of Books Converging Chinese and Western Medicine***, Zhu Peiwen (About in the middle of the 19th century) and his ***Treatise on Illustrations of Internal Organs Both in Chinese and Western Medicine,*** Zhang Xichun (1860—1933 A.D.) and his ***Records of Traditional Chinese and Western Medicine in Combination*** and so on. Today most Chinese !medical scholars advocate that Chinese, Western and Combined medicines should advance together and exist side by side for a long time. As a matter of fact, Chinese and Western medicines are two medical sciences with different theoretical systems developed under different historical conditions. They are both the fruit of prolonged hard work, intelligence and wisdom of all mankind. Either of them has merits and shortcomings. Yet both have human beings as the object of study. Hence they should cooperate with and learn from each other, learning from the other's strong points to offset its own weaknesses. It is predictable that Chinese medicine and Western medicine will gradually merge into a single entity partly because of the rapid advance of the world's science and technology and partly because of the steady development of Chinese medicine and Western medicine in practice and theory, and their renewal and mutual osmosis as well. mankind will enjoy this new type of medicine in the future.

Traditional Chinese medicine has now reached a new stage

近百年来，随着西医在中国广泛地传播，形成中医、西医并存的局面。不少医家逐渐认识到中西医各有所长，因此试图把两种学术加以汇通，并从理论到临床提出了一系列汇通中西医的见解，逐渐形成了中西医汇通思潮与学派。其代表人物及其著作是：唐宗海(公元1862～1918)之《中西汇通医书五种》；朱沛文(约19世纪中期)之《华洋脏腑图像合纂》；张锡纯（公元1860～1933)之《医学衷中参西录》等。当今中国学者多主张中医、西医、中西医结合医长期并存，共同发展。事实上，中医、西医是在不同历史条件下发展起来的两种不同理论体系的医学科学，都是人类长期辛勤劳动、聪明才智的结晶，各有所长，亦各有所短。但其研究对象都是人。中西医应密切合作，互相学习，取长补短。可以预言，伴随着世界科学技术相关学科的突飞猛进，以及中西医各自在实践、理论上的不断发展、更新与相互渗透，二者必然会逐渐融为一体，贡献于人类。

目前中医学已进入了新的发展阶段。1986年1月4日中华

of development. On January 4, 1986, the State Council of the People's Republic of China decreed that the State Administrative Bureau of TCM and Pharmacy be established. This leading body exercises control over TCM and Chinese materia medica, the step-by-step combination of Chinese and Western medicine as well as the medical teaching and research work of national medicine and pharmacy throughout China.

In China, with regard to TCM, there are, now, 340,000 doctors, 1,500 hospitals with 100,000 beds, 26 colleges and 30 academies. In TCM researches, great importance has been attached not only to the systematization and compilation of the documents of various ages, but also to the application of modern scientific approaches in carrying out researches in terms of the basic theories of TCM. As a result, much improvement has been made in the treatment of common diseases, frequently encountered diseases and difficult and complicated cases.

From what has been said above, it is not hard to see that TCM is a traditional medicine which has a long history, high practical value and boundless prospects. It is worth learning, studying and applying all over the world.

Section 2

Basic Characteristics of TCM

TCM has many characteristics both in the understanding of the human body's physiology and pathology and in the diagnosis and treatment of diseases. These characteristics, however, can be summarized in the following two aspects:

1. The Concept of the Organism as a Whole

By "organic whole" we mean entirety and unity. TCM

人民共和国国务院决定成立国家中医药管理局，统管全国的中医药、中西医结合和民族医药的医、教、研工作。

全国现在有中医34万人，中医医院1,500所，病床100,000张，高等中医院校26所，中等中医学校30所。中医科研一方面加强了对中医历代文献的整理研究，另一方面亦开始采用现代科学的方法研究中医的基本理论，并在治疗常见病、多发病以及疑难病方面取得了一定进展。

由上不难看出，中医学是一门既有悠久历史，又有较高实用价值，并有广阔前途，值得世界人民共同学习、研究和应用的传统医学。

第二节　中医学的基本特点

中医学在对人体生理、病理的认识以及在疾病的诊断和治疗方面有许多特点，但概而言之，不外以下两个方面：

1. 整体观念

整体，就是完整性、统一性。中医学十分重视人体本身的统

attaches great importance to the unity of the human body itself and its relationship with nature, and holds that the human body itself is an organic whole and has very close and inseparable relations with the external natural surroundings. The concept of emphasizing the unity within the body and the unified relations between the body and the outside world is known as that of an organic whole.

1) The Unity within the Body

The human body is made up of viscera, bowels, tissues and other organs. Each of them has its own special physiological functions. All these different physiological functions are a component part of the entire life process of the body. And this determines the unity within the body. Therefore, the component parts of the human body are inseparable from each other in structure, related, subsidiary and conditonal to each other in physiology, and of certain influence upon each other in pathology. These mutual relations and influences are centered around the five viscera (the heart, the liver, the spleen, the lung and the kidney) and come into effect through the channels and collaterals. For instance, the heart is interior-exteriorly related to the small intestine, controls blood circulation ,and has its "specific opening" in the tongue proper and so on. Look at the folloing table:

Five Viscera	Six Bowels	Five Body Constituents (body tissues)	Five Sense Organs (external organs)	Remarks
heart	small intestine	vessel	tongue	Of the six bowels the triple warmer doesn't coordinate with the five viscera. In the
lung	large intestine	skin	nose	

一性及其与自然界的相互关系，认为人体本身是一个有机的整体，人体与外界自然环境有着密切的、不可分割的联系。这种既强调人体内部的统一性，又重视人体与外界环境统一性的观念，被称之为整体观念。

1）人体内部的统一性

人体是由若干脏腑、组织和器官所组成的，它们有各自不同的生理功能，而这些不同的生理功能又都是整体活动的一个组成部分，这就决定了人体内部的统一性。因此，人体各个组成部分之间，在结构上是不可分割的，在生理上是相互联系、相互资助、相互制约的，在病理上也是相互影响的。这种相互联系、相互影响，是以五脏为中心，通过经络的联络作用而实现的。如心合小肠、主血脉、开窍于舌……等，具体见下表：

五　脏	六　腑	五　体（形体组织）	五　官（外部器官）	备　注
心	小　肠	脉	舌	六腑中还有三焦，不与五脏配合。
肺	大　肠	皮	鼻	

spleen	stomach	muscle	mouth	in the theory of channels and collaterals, they and the pericardium channel are interior-exteriorly related.
liver	gallbladder	tendon	eye	
kidney	urinary bladder	bone	ear, the two (front and back) private parts, i.e., urethral orifice and anus	

2) The Unity between the Human Body and Nature

Man lives in nature and takes nature as his vital conditions for living. In the meantime, he is influenced directly or indirectly by the movements and changes in nature, to which he is bound to make corresponding physiological and pathological responses. For example, as the climate varies with the four seasons in a year, the normal pulse conditions (including pulse rate, rhythm, volume, tension, etc.) are also varied. The pulse becomes string-like in spring, full in summer, floating in autumn and sunken in winter. This provides a basis for doctors to distinguish abnormal pulse conditions from the normal ones during the clinical diagnosis. The occurence, development and changes of many diseases are seasonal. For example, spring witnesses more epidemic febrile diseases; summer more sunstrokes; autumn more cases with symptoms of dryness and winter more cold-stroke syndromes. Of course, people can certainly reduce or eliminate some seasonal diseases by doing physical exercises, transforming nature and taking active measures of prevention. TCM physicians also have observed that along with alternation of early morning, late afternoon, daytime and night in a day, a disease may become severer or

脾	胃	肉	口	
肝	胆	筋	目	在经络学说中与
肾	膀胱	骨	耳、前后三阴	心包络配为表里
				关系

2）人与自然界的统一性

人类生活在自然界，以自然界为其生存的必要条件。同时，自然界的运动变化又可直接或间接地影响着人体，而人体也必然相应地产生生理或病理上的反映。例如：由于一年四季的气候不同，正常脉象就有春弦、夏洪、秋浮、冬沉的变化，这就为医生在临床诊断时鉴别常脉与病脉提供了依据；许多疾病的发生、发展与变化，有着明显的季节性。如春季多温病，夏季多中暑，秋季多燥症，冬季多伤寒。当然，人们通过锻炼身体，改造自然，积极预防，又可减少或消除某些季节性疾病。中医还观察到，一

milder. For instance, the monograph entitled Regarding a Day as a Year Consisting of the Four Seasons, a chapter of Miraculous Pivot) says, "There are various diseases, most of which become milder in the morning, better during the daytime, worse again in the late afternoon and even severer at night". This because "In the morning the vital energy of the human body begins to grow stronger, while the pathogenic factors weaker; at midday the vital energy of the human body is predominant and lords it over the pathogenic factors; in the late afternoon the vital energy of the human body begins to become weaker, while the pathogenic factors stronger; at midnight, the vital energy of the human body returns to the internal organs, while the pathogenic factors come into leading place". In modern times, someone has also noticed that human pulse conditions, temperature, the amount of oxygen consumed, carbon dioxide released and hormone secreted have biorhythms during the 24 hours of a day. This finding may promote the round-the-clock exploration of the physiological and pathological changes of the human body.

Based on the theory of the circulaton of *qi* characteristics of TCM, the pathogenesis of the human body is often influenced by the periodic changes of the climate, which take place every 12 years or every sixty years. In recent years, scientists have realized that the law of these periodic changes has something to do with the cycle of sunspots, which is formed every 11 to 12 years. Their movements bring about periodic changes in the radiation of sunlight, interfere with the magnetic field of the earth, and change the climate around the earth, thus exerting impact upon the physiology and pathology of the human body.

TCM believes that different geographical surroundings produce different effects on the physiology and pathology of the human body. The effects are even so great as to extend or shorten human lives. For instance, On Conventions of the

日中朝、夕、昼、夜的变化，亦可影响疾病的轻重，如《灵枢·顺气一日分为四时篇》云："夫百病者，多以旦慧昼安，夕加夜甚。"其机理，是因为"朝则人气始生，病气衰；日中人气长，长则胜邪。夕则人气始衰，邪气始生；夜半人气入脏，邪气独居于身"。近代有人亦观察到，人的脉搏、体温、耗氧量、二氧化碳的释放量、激素的分泌等，都具有24小时节律。这对探讨人体昼夜生理、病理的变化，可能有所帮助。

中医特有的运气学说认为，气候有着十二年、六十年的周期变化，因而人体的发病也常受其影响。近年来，科学家们发现这种十二年或六十年的变化规律与太阳黑子活动周期有关。太阳黑子的活动周期为十一至十二年，它的活动会使太阳光辐射产生周期性变化，并强烈干扰地磁，改变气候，从而对人体的生理、病理产生影响。

中医学认为，不同的地理环境对人体的生理、病理亦有不同影响，甚至影啊到人的寿命。如《素问·五常政大论》说："高者其

Five Circuit Phases, a chapter of ***Plain Questions*** says: "People who live in the high areas have a long life, while those who live in the low ones die young. Living areas differ in altitude. A little difference in height causes a little difference in life, while a great difference in height results in a great difference in life. Therefore, physicians have to know the law of nature and geographical conditions". Modern researches have shown that the mountain area between 1,500 and 2,000 metres above the sea level is the ideal geographical surroundings for a long life, because it is a place where hydrogen anions are concentrated.

3) The Guiding Function of the Concept of the Organism as a Whole

The concept of the organism as a whole not only embodies TCM's understanding of the human body itself and the relationship between it and nature, but also provides the medical workers with a necessary method of thinking in treating diseases. Such a concept penetrates through the entire theory concerning the physiology and pathology of TCM, and of great significance in guiding diagnosis and treatment. For example, TCM believes "The heart has its specific opening in the tongue proper", so the physiological functions and pathological changes of the heart can be known by observing the tongue. Pale tongue indicates the blood deficiency of the heart; purple tongue with petechiae, the blood stagnation of the heart. To cure these diseases, the first important thing of all is to find out where the key pathogenesis is according to the relationship between the heart and the tongue, by taking into consideration of the concept of the organism as a whole, and by making a comprehensive analysis of the case. Another example, acupuncture therapies of TCM, *Zi Wu Liu Zhu* (select the acupoint on the basis of "five *shu* points" of the twelve channels matching the "heavenly stems and earthly branches") and *Ling Gui Ba Fa* (select the acupoint according to the eight

气寿，下者其气夭，地之小大异也，小者小异，大者大异。故治病者，必明天道地理……。”现代研究证实，海拔1,500至2,000米之间的山区，氢负离子密集，确是长寿的地理环境。

3）整体观念的指导意义

整体观念是中医学对人体本身、人与自然界相互关系的认识，也是中医工作者诊治疾病时所必须具备的思想方法。它贯穿于中医的生理、病理之中，对诊断和治疗具有重要的指导意义。如中医学认为，“心开窍于舌”，通过望舌可以测知心脏的生理功能与病理变化。心血不足，可见舌质淡白；心血瘀阻，可见舌紫或有瘀点……。治疗时就应根据心与舌的关系，从整体观念出发，全

points in the eight extra-channels matching the "heavenly stems and earthly branches"), have obvious curative effects just because the acupoints and acutime are determined according to the relationship between the working of the channels, pulse, vital energy and blood of the human body on one side and time on the other. The most adequate time should be also chosen for taking herbal medicines. For instance, Ten Jujube Decoction, *Shi Zao Tang* in the book ***Treatise on Febrile Diseases*** written by Zhang Zhongjing in 219 A.D. is better to be taken on an empty stomach in the early morning; Cock Crowing Powder, *Ji Ming San* which is recorded in the book ***Standards for Diagnosis and Treatment*** by Wang Kentang in 1,602 A.D. should be taken at daybreak when cocks begin to crow. Modern medicine has also noticed that the effect of digital is taken by the patient with heart failure at about 4 o'clock in the early morning is 40 times greater than that of it taken at any other time. And insuline, if taken at the time mentioned above, is most effective for the patients with diabetes, too.

Why does the human body have such a close relationship with nature, and why does the human body itself act in accordance with such a strict time rhythm and regularity ? In recent years, some scholars have pointed out that these result both from the adaptation of all living things to the changes of physical surroundings such as the earth's revolution,rotation and so on,and from the domination of some structure within the body. Now it has been proved that in the nucleus suprachiasmaticus (SCH), epiphysis, pituitary bodies and adrenal gland, there exist such structures as to control the time rhythm and regularity. From the foregoing it is easy to see that the concept of "*Tian Ren Xiang Ying*" (relevant adaptation of the human body to natural environment in TCM) has its material base and a scientific basis as well.

面分析病情，找出关键病机之所在而治之。再如中医的子午流注、灵龟八法之针刺疗法，就是根据人体经脉气血的时间节律，确定针刺穴位和针刺时间，其疗效显著。某些中药的服用，亦需选择一个最佳时间。如《伤寒论》之十枣汤，宜在平旦服，即清晨(空腹)服；《证治准绳》之鸡鸣散，须在清晨鸡鸣时服。现代医学亦观察到，心力衰竭患者在清晨4时左右时服洋地黄，其疗效大于平时服40倍；糖尿病患者清晨4时左右时服胰岛素，亦最敏感。

为什么人与自然界有如此密切的关系，人体本身又有如此严格的时间节律呢？近年来不少学者指出，这是因为各种生物在其漫长的进化过程中，为适应地球的公转与自转等物理环境变化，并受体内某一结构控制而产生的。现已证明，人的下丘脑视交叉上核、松果体、脑垂体和肾上腺，都有调节时间节律的结构。由此可见，中医的“天人相应”观确有其物质基础和科学依据。

2. Diagnosis and Treatment Based on an Overall Analysis of Signs and Symptoms

By "*Bian Zheng*" we mean analysing the relevant information, signs and symptoms collected through the four methods of diagnosis (observation, listening and smelling, inquiring, pulse feeling and palpation) in the light of the theory of TCM, having a good idea of the cause, nature and location of a disease, and the relationship between pathogenic factors and the vital energy, and summarizing them into "*Zheng*" of a certain nature (syndrome). By "*Shi Zhi*" we mean determining the corresponding therapeutic method according to the conclusion of an overall differentiation of symptoms, signs and others.

In clinical treatment, TCM physicians do not focus their main attention on the similarities and dissimilarities between diseases but on the differences between the syndromes they have. Generally speaking, the same syndromes are treated in similar ways, while different syndromes are treated in different ways. Take cold for example, if it manifests itself in more severe chilliness, slight fever, a tongue with thin and white fur then it belongs to the exterior syndrome caused by wind and cold, and should be treated with strong sudorific drugs pungent in taste and warm in property, to dispel the wind and cold; if its manifestations are more severe fever, milder chilliness, a tongue with thin and yellow fur, then it belongs to the exterior syndrome caused by wind and heat, and should be treated with mild diaphoretics pungent in taste and cool in property, to dispel the wind and heat. This is called "treating the same diseases with different methods". Sometimes, different diseases have same syndromes in nature, so their treatments are basically the same. If clinical analysis and differentiation show that persistent dysentery, prolapse of the rectum, uterus and others belong to the syndrome of "sinking

2. 辨证施治

所谓"辨证"，就是将四诊(望、闻、问、切)所收集的有关资料、症状和体征，运用中医的理论加以分析，辨清疾病的病因、性质、部位以及邪正关系，判断为某种性质的"证"所谓"施治"，又称"论治"，就是根据辨证的结果，确定相应的治疗方法。

中医治病主要不是着眼于"病"的异同，而是着眼于"证"的区别。相同的证，用基本相同的治法；不同的证，用基本不同的治法。以感冒为例，如表现为恶寒重、发热轻、舌苔薄白，属风寒表证，治疗用辛温解表法；如表现为发热重、恶寒轻、舌苔薄黄，属风热表证，治疗则用辛凉解表法。此即所谓"同病异治"。有时不同的病可以出现同一性质的证，治疗时同样采用基本相同的治

of the *qi*" (functional activities of the middle warmer, the middle portion of the body cavity housing the spleen and stomach), then their treating method should be the same one, lifting the *qi* of the middle warmer. This is called "treating different diseases with the same method".

In China, quite a number of colleges of medicine and pharmacy and scientific research institutes are undertaking the researches on the esssence of "*Zheng*" (syndrome) in TCM. For example, Chongqing Medical College holds that "*Zheng*" is the comprehensive manifestation of the disorderly relations, resulting from the pathogen and pathogenic condition between the whole body and its reactive characteristics on one side and its surroundings (including nature and society) on the other, between viscera, bowels, channels and collaterals, between cells themselves and between cells and body fluid; that "*Zheng*" is a reaction of life substances characterized by time-phase and essentiality in the course of a disease; and that "*Zheng*" is a whole-finalized pattern of reaction which mainly manifests itself in the clinical functional changes. Other scholars believe, from the point of vague mathematics, that "*Zheng*" is a vague collectivity made up of such materials as symptoms, signs and characteristics.

Of course diagnosis and treatment based on an overall analysis and differentiation of symptoms and signs should not remain at the present level or stand still or refuse to make any further progress, but instead, be enriched, renewed, developed and improved continually alongside the advancing of modern natural sciences.

法。如久痢、脱肛、子宫脱垂等，如通过辨析均属“中气下陷”证，治疗都采用“升提中气”法，此即所谓“异病同治”。

关于中医“证”实质的研究，中国不少医药院校和科研机构正在着手进行。如重庆医学院认为，证是机体在致病原因和条件作用下所发生的整体体质反应特征和整体与周围环境(包括自然、社会)之间、脏腑经络与脏腑经络之间，细胞与细胞之间，细胞与体液之间相互关系紊乱的综合表现；证是生命物质在疾病过程中具有时相性、本质性的反应；是一种以临床机能变化为主的“整体定型反应形式”。有的学者则从模糊数学角度认为，证是由症状、体征和特征等信息组成的模糊集合。

当然，辨证施治不应停留在原有的水平上固步自封，而应随着现代自然科学的进步不断地充实、更新、发展和提高。

Chapter Two

The Theory of *Yin* and *Yang* As Well As Five Elements

What is *yin* and *yang* ? *yin* and *yang* means the two fundamental principles or forces in the universe, ever opposing and supplementing each other. It is an ancient philosophical concept used in traditional Chinese medicine (TCM). As to the concept of the five elements, it refers to wood, fire, earth, metal and water, each having its own special properties. This is also taken as one of the ancient philosophical concepts used in TCM.

Section 1

The Theory of *Yin* and *Yang*

1. The Formation of the Theory of *Yin* and *Yang*

Yin and *yang* was originally included in the category of the ancient philosophy of China. At first, *yin* and *yang* meant whether a place faces the sun or not. The place being exposed to the sun is *yang*, whereas the place not having a southern exposure is *yin*. The southern side of a mountain, for example, is *yang*, while the northern side of it is *yin*. Subsequently, through long-term living, practice and observation of every kind of natural phenomenon, people have come to realize that *yin* and *yang*, the two components which oppose each other, exist in all things, and that, furthermore, their interaction

第 二 章

阴阳五行学说

何谓阴阳？阴阳意指万物中始终相互对立、相互资生的两个基本方面。它是一个古老的哲学概念，并被中医所应用。至于五行，则是指木、火、土、金、水，它们各有其独自的特性，也是被中医所应用的古代哲学概念之一。

第一节　阴阳学说

1.阴阳学说的形成

阴阳，本属中国古代哲学的范畴。最初，阴阳是指日光的向背，即向日光的地方为阳，背日光的地方为阴。如山南为阳，山北为阴。后来，人们通过长期的生活、实践和对各种自然现象的观察，逐渐发现事物都普遍存在着相互对立的阴阳两个方面，进而认识到两者的相互作用促进了事物的发生、发展与转化，因而

promotes the occurrence, development and transformation of things. In consequence *yin* and *yang* is used as the means of reasoning things out in analysing all the phenomena in the natural world. "*Lao Zi*", a philosophical work written in ancient China, says: "All things on earth carry *yin* on their backs and hold *yang* in their arms." That is, each thing contains the two components of *yin* and *yang*. "*Zhou Yi*", also an ancient philosophical work, draws from the complicated natural and social phenomena the same two philosophical concepts, *yin* and *yang*, whose symbols are (- -) and (—), and advocates *yin* and *yang* as the "*Dao*" (the basic law in the natural world) of the heaven and earth, that is, to consider the transformation of *yin* and *yang* into each other as the basic law in the universe.

The impact of *yin* and *yang* theory on the science of TCM has promoted the formation and development of TCM's own theoretical system and, finally it, itself, becomes an important component part of the dasic theory of TCM.

2. The Content of the Theory of *Yin* and *Yang*

The content of the theory of *yin* and *yang* can be described briefly as follows: opposition, interdependence, relative waxing and wanning, and transformation.

1) Opposition and Interdependence of *Yin* and *Yang*

By the opposition of *yin* and *yang*, we mean all things and phenomena in the natural world contain the two opposite components. For example, the heaven and earth, outside and inside, movement and stability, coming in and going out, day and night, cold and heat, rising and falling, etc., all these are opposites. In the theory of *yin* and *yang*, the heaven is considered as *yang*, while the earth is *yin*; outside is *yang*, while inside is *yin*; movement is *yong*, while stabilty is yin; going out is *yang* while comingin is *yin*; day is *yang*, while night is *yin*; heat is *yang*, while cold is *yin*; rising is *yang*, while falling is *yin*; rapid pulse is *yang*,

就以阴阳为说理工具来解释自然界的各种现象。如中国古代的一部哲学著作《老子》所说“万物负阴而抱阳”，即认为一切事物都包含着阴和阳两个方面。《周易》也是一部古代哲学著作。它从复杂的自然现象和社会现象中抽象出“阴”和“阳”两个相对的哲学概念，其符号为(- -)和(—)，并提出“一阴一阳之谓道”，即把阴阳交替看作宇宙的根本规律。

阴阳学说对中医学的影响，促进了中医理论体系的形成与发展，最后，它本身也成了中医基本理论的一个重要组成部分。

2.阴阳学说的内容

阴阳学说的内容可以用“对立、互根、消长、转化”来概括。

1）对立、互根

阴阳对立，是指自然界的一切事物和现象，都存在着相互对立的两个方面，如天与地、内与外、动与静、出与入、昼与夜、寒与热、升与降等。阴阳学说认为：天为阳，地为阴；外为阳，内为阴；动为阳，静为阴；出为阳，入为阴；昼为阳，夜为阴；热为阳，寒为阴；升为阳，降为阴；脉数为阳，脉迟为阴等。都

while slow pulse is *yin*. These opposite pairs show that *yin* and *yang* exist within all things and phenomena.

Yin and *yang* not only oppose but also contain each other, without the other, neither can exist. For instance, there would be no earth without heaven, and vice versa. Without outside, there would be no inside, and vice versa. This relationship of coexistence is known as interdepencence. TCM holds that "functional movement" belongs to *yang*, "nourishing substance" to *yin*, and that the one can not exist without the other; for example, if the intestines and other internal organs do not move, "nourishing substance" can not be digested or absorbed; and if over a long period "nourishing substances" are not provided, the organs cease to move. The book, ***Canon of Medicne*** (722—221 B.C.), says: "*Yin* in the interior is the guardian of *yang*, *yang* in the exterior is the activator of *yin*". This also shows the relationship of interdependence between *yin* and *yang*.

2) The Waxing and Waning of *Yin* and *Yang*, and the Transformation between *Yin* and *Yang*

What is meant by the waxing and waning of *yin* and *yang*? *Yin* and *yang* opposing each other and yet depending on each other for existence, are not stagnant but in a dynamic state, i.e., while *yin* wanes, *yang* waxes, and vice versa. This dynamic change of succeeding each other between *yin* and *yang* is known as the waxing and waning of *yin* and *yang*. Take the seasonal climatic variations in the natural world for example. The weather gets warm when winter gives way to spring, and hot when spring gives way to summer, during which time *yin* wanes, while *yang* waxes. However, it gets cool when autumn replaces summer, and cold when winter replaces autumn in which time *yang* wanes, but *yin* waxes.

By "transformation" we mean *yin* and *yang* will transform into each other under certain conditions. For instance, in the course of suffering from a disease, the patient runs a high fever,

说明阴阳的对立普遍存在于一切事物和现象之中。

阴阳两方面既是对立的，又是相互依存的，任何一方都不能脱离另一方面单独存在。如没有天就无所谓地，没有地也就无所谓天；没有外就无所谓内，没有内也就无所谓外……。阴阳这种相互依存关系，称之为阴阳互根。中医认为："功能活动"属阳，"营养物质"属阴，它们中的任何一方都不能脱离另一方面而单独存在。例如，如果小肠和其他内脏器官不能发挥其作用，"营养物质"就不能消化、吸收；反之，如"营养物质"长期得不到供给，器官的功能就会停止。《内经》云："阴在内，阳之守也；阳在外，阴之使也"，亦为阴阳互根的例证。

2)消长、转化

阴阳消长，是说，相互对立、相互依存的双方不是静止不变的，而是处于动态变化之中，即处于"阴消阳长"、"阳消阴长"互为消长的变化之中。阴阳之间的这种彼此消长的动态变化称之为阴阳消长。以自然界四季的气候变化为例，从冬至春至夏，气候由寒变温变热，即为"阴消阳长"的过程，而由夏至秋至冬，气候由热变凉变寒，则为"阳消阴长"的过程。

阴阳转化，是说阴阳双方在一定条件下可以相互转化。例如，

has a red complexion, feels irritable and restless, and gets into a rapid and strong pulse condition. But all of a sudden, he feels listless, his temperature becomes lower, his face turns pale, and his pulse condition becomes so fine that the pulse is almost cut off. This is an example of transformation between *yin* and *yang*.

The general law according to which things are distinguished into *yin* or *yang* is as follows. All that are hyperfunctional, excited, hot, moving, strong, bright, invisible. light and clear, up and upwards, out and outwards, and all that have active specific characteristics belong to *yang*. On the contrary, all that are waning, restricted, cold, weak, dark, visible, heavy and turbid, down and downwards, in and inwards and all that have inactive specific characteristics belong to *yin*. It should be pointed out that the *yin* or *yang* property of things is not absolute but relative. This relativity of *yin* and *yang* is shown in the intertransformation between *yin* and *yang* mentioned above, i.e, *yin* may transform into *yang* and vice versa; it is also shown in the constant divisibility of *yin* and *yang*, i.e., either *yin* or *yang* can be still divided into another pair of *yin* and *yang*. For instance, day is of *yang* nature and night is of *yin* nature, but both day and night can be again divided like this: the period from dawn till noon is the *yang* aspect of *yang*; the period from noon till dusk is the *yin* aspect of *yang*; the period from dusk till midnight is the *yin* aspect of *yin*; the period from midnight till dawn is the *yang* aspect of *yin*.

3. Uses of the Theory of *Yin* and *Yang* in TCM

Yin and *yang* is embodied in every aspect of TCM's theoretical system. It is used to explain the tissues and structures, physiology and pathology of the human body, and direct clinical diagnosis and treatment.

1) Using *Yin* and *Yang* to Explain the Tissues and Structures of the Human Body

According to the theory of *yin* and *yang*, it is considered

在疾病过程中，高热、面赤、烦燥、脉数有力的病人突然转为精神萎靡、体温下降、面色苍白、脉微欲绝，就是阴阳转化的例证。

事物分属阴阳的一般规律是：凡是亢进的、兴奋的、热的、动的、强壮的、光明的、无形的、轻清的、在上向上的在外向外的……等具有积极特性的事物，都属于阳；与此相反，凡是衰退的、抑制的、冷的、静的、虚弱的、晦暗的、有形的、重浊的、在下向下的、在内向内的……等具有消极特性的事物，都属于阴。需要指出的是：事物的阴阳属性不是绝对的，而是相对的。这种相对性既表现为上面所提到的“阴阳转化”，如阴可以转化为阳，阳亦可转化为阴；又表现在阴阳的无限可分性，即阴阳之中仍可再分阴阳。如昼为阳，夜为阴，但昼和夜还可这样再分：上午为阳中之阳，下午为阳中之阴；前半夜为阴中之阴，后半夜为阴中之阳。

3.阴阳学说在中医学中的应用

阴阳学说贯穿在中医理论体系的各个方面，并以此来解释人体的组织结构、生理病理，并指导着临床诊断和治疗。

1)说明人体的组织结构

that opposite but unitive phenomena between *yin* and *yang* exist between rostral and caudal, inside and outside, exterior and interior, dorsal and ventral aspects of every tissue and structure of the human body. When speaking of *yin* and *yang* in the human body, the upper part is *yang*, the lower part *yin*; the exterior is *yang*, the interior *yin*; the back is *yang*, the abdomen *yin*; the lateral aspect of the extremities is *yang*; the medial aspect *yin*. When speaking of *yin* and *yang* of the internal organs in the body, the five viscera, i.e., the heart, liver, spleen, lung and kidney, are *yin*, because their functions of preserving vital substance tend to be stable; the six bowels organs, i.e., the gallbladder, stomach, large intestine, small intestine, urinary bladder and triple warmer, are *yang*, because their functions of transmitting and digesting water and food tend to be active. The relationship between *yin* and *yang* also remains constant among the five viscera. The heart and lung are *yang*, because of being higher, while the liver, spleen and kidney are *yin*, because of being lower. When speaking of *yin* and *yang* of every organ, the function is *yang*, the substance *yin*. When speaking of *yin* and *yang* of the channels and collaterals, the channels may be divided into channels belonging to *yin* and channels belonging to *yang*. Collaterals can also be classified as *yin* collaterals and *yang* collaterals. When speaking of *yin* and *yang* of the twelve channels, three are *yang* channels of the hand and three *yin* channels of the hand, three *yang* channels of the foot and three *yin* channels of the foot. As to the vital energy and blood, vital energy (*qi*) is *yang*, blood *yin*.

2) Using *Yin* ang *Yang* to Explain the Physiological Function of the Human Body

TCM believes that the normal physiological functions of the human body result from the opposite, unitive and coordinate relation between *yang* (function) and *yin* (substance). *Yin* and *yang* are always in the state of dynamic balance. It is

阴阳学说认为，人体上下、内外、表里、前后各组织结构之间，以及每一组织结构本身，无不包含着阴阳对立统一现象。就人体部位而言，人体的上部属阳，下部属阴；体表属阳，体内属阴；背部属阳，腹部属阴；四肢的外侧属阳，内侧属阴。就人体脏腑而言，五脏即心、肺、脾、肝、肾属阴（因其贮藏精气的功能偏于静），六腑即胆、胃、大肠、小肠、膀胱、三焦属阳（因其传化水谷的功能偏于动）。五脏之中还可再分阴阳，即心、肺居上属阳，肝、脾、肾居下属阴。且就每一脏器来说，功能为阳，物质为阴。就经络而言，经可分为阴经、阳经，络又可分为阴络、阳络；就十二经脉而言，即有手三阳经与手三阴经之分，足三阳经与足三阴经之别。就气血而言，气为阳，血为阴。

2）说明人体的生理功能

中医学认为，人体的正常生理活动是阳（功能）与阴（物质）保持对立、统一的协调关系的结果，阴阳总是处于动态平衡状态中，

known as "*yin* is even and well while *yang* is firm, hence a relative equilibrium is maintained and health is guaranteed". Physiological function is based on substance. Without substance, including the essence of life, blood, constructive energy and body fluid, there would be no source for functions. But the metabolism of substance must depend on the performance of function. If *yin* and *yang* of the human body separate from each other and can not aid each other, life will come to an end. This is what is called, in TCM, "the divorce of *yin* and *yang* means the end of one's life."

3) Using *Yin* and *Yang* to Explain the Pathological Changes of the Human Body

In TCM, it is thought that the imbalance of *yin* and *yang* is one of the basic pathogeneses of a disease. For example, preponderance of *yang* leads to hyperfunction of the organism and heat manifestations, while preponderance of *yin* hypofunction of the organism or endogenous cold. Deficiency of *yang* brings on symptoms of external cold, while deficiency of *yin* as the result of exhausted vital essence leads to endogenous heat. *Yang* in excess makes *yin* suffer, while *yin* in excess makes *yang* suffer. In severe damage of *yang*, *yin* is involved, in severe damage of *yin*, *yang* is involved, too. Thus, *yin* and *yang* are both damaged. A case of *yin* nature (hypofunction) in its extreme may show *yang* (hyperfunction) symptoms and signs, while a case of *yang* nature (hyperfunction) in its extreme will give rise to *yin* (hypofunction) symptoms and signs.

4) Using *Yin* and *Yang* to Diagnose and Treat Diseases

Because one of the basic pathogeneses of a disease is the imbalance of *yin* and *yang*, any disease, no matter how intricate and volatile its clinical manifestations, can be diagnosed with the theory of *yin* and *yang*. Although diseases are classified as

中医称之为“阴平阳秘，精神乃治”。生理功能是以物质为基础的，没有物质(包括精、血、营、津液等)，就无从产生功能；而物质代谢又必须依赖功能活动才能完成。若人体的阴阳不能相互为用而分离，人的生命也就终止了。此即中医所说的“阴阳离决，精神乃绝”。

3)说明人体的病理变化

中医学认为，人体阴阳失调是疾病发生的基本病机之一。如阳盛则热，阴盛则寒；阳虚生外寒，阴虚生内热；阳盛则阴病，阴盛则阳病；阳损及阴，阴损及阳，阴阳俱损；重阴必阳，重阳必阴等。

4)用于诊断和治疗

由于疾病的基本病机之一就是阴阳失调，所以任何疾病，尽管其临床表现错综复杂、千变万化，都可用阴阳学说来诊断。如

exterior and interior according to their locations, and as cold, heat, asthenia and sthenia according to their nature, if the theory of *yin* and *yang* is used, the types of exterior, heat and sthenia are *yang*; interior, cold and asthenia *yin*. In TCM, in making a diagnosis, the first important thing is to ascertain whether the disease is *yin* or *yang*. For example in observation of the patients' complexion, those who look bright are patients of the *yang* character, while those who look dark and gloomy are patients of the *yin* character. In listening and smelling, those who have a loud and clear voice have a *yang* character, while those who have a low and weak voice a *yin* character. In inquiring, those who have a fever, feel thirsty, suffer from constipation and have a rapid pulse condition are of *yang*, while those who have an aversion to cold, don't feel thirsty, have loose stools and a slow pulse condition are of *yin*. In pulse feeling and palpation, those whose pulses are floating, rapid, large, slippery and full are of *yang*, while those whose pulses are deep, slow, small, rough and empty are of *yin*.

How is the theory of *yin* and *yang* used in treating diseases in TCM? Preponderance of *yang* leads to hyperfunction of the organism and heat manifestations, which is known as sthenic heat syndrome. In treating sthenic heat syndrome, drugs of cold and cool nature should be used in order to inhibit the preponderance of *yang*, i.e., heat syndrme must be treated with drugs cold in nature. Preponderance of *yin* leads to hypofunction of the organism or endogenous cold which is called cold-sthenia syndrome. In treating it, drugs of a warm-heat nature should be used so as to restrict the predominance of *yin*, i.e., cold syndrome should be treated with drugs warm in property. The deficiency of *yang* brings on symptoms of external cold, which are called deficiency-cold syndrome. In treating it, drugs of warm and invigorating nature should be used. This is known as treating the hyperactivity of *yin* by supplementing *yang*, the source of fire. The deficiency of

病位有表、里之分，病性有寒、热、虚、实之别，若用阴阳来归纳，则表、热、实属阳，里、寒、虚属阴。中医诊断疾病，首先要分清阴阳。如望诊：色泽鲜明者属阴，晦暗者属阴；闻诊，声音洪亮者属阳，低微无力者属阴；问诊：发热、口渴、便秘、脉数属阳，恶寒、口不渴、便溏、脉迟者属阴；切诊：脉浮、数、大、滑、实者属阳，沉、迟、小、涩、虚者属阴。

如何在治疗疾病时运用阴阳学说呢？对阳盛则热的实热证，宜用寒凉药以抑其阳，即"热者寒之"；对阴盛则寒的寒实证，宜用温热药以制其阴，即"寒者热之"；对"阳虚生外寒"的虚寒证，

yin as a result of exhausted vital essence leads to endogenous heat, which is called as asthenic heat syndrome. In treating it drugs of nourishing *yin* should be used. This is what is known, in TCM, as replenishing the vital essence, (especially that of the kidney and liver) to check virtual *yang* (exuberance of the vital function) caused by the deficiency of *yin* factor. In treating those diseases in which there is severe damage of *yang*, *yin* is involved, although the first thing is to reinforce the vital function, yet, the vital essence, at the same time, should be also invigorated. In treating those diseases in which there is severe damage of *yin*, *yang* is involved, while the vital essence is being replenished, the vital function should be strengthened, too. In treating those diseases resulting from the deficiency of both *yin* and *yang*, both the vital essence and the vital function should be replenished.

The property, flavour and function of Chinese medicinal herbs can also be summarized in the light of the *yin* and *yang* theory, and this forms a basis for the clinical application of Chinese medicinal herbs. For example, the herbs of cold and cool nature belong to *yin*; while the herbs warm and hot in nature, *yang*. The herbs with sour, bitter and salty flavours belong to *yin*, while the herbs with pungent, sweet and bland flavours, *yang*. The herbs with astringent and subsiding function belong to *yin*, while the herbs with dispersing, ascending and floating function, *yang*. In TCM, the principles of treatment are established just on the basis of the predominance or weakness of *yin* and *yang*. Once the principle is established, herbs are selected according to their property of *yin* and *yang* and their function. In so doing, one can achieve the aim of curing diseases.

宜用温补药，即“益火之源，以消阴翳”；对阴虚生内热的虚热证，宜用滋阴药，即“壮水之主，以制阳光”；对阳损及阴的，在补阳的同时兼顾益阴；阴损及阳的，在补阴的同时兼顾扶阳；阴阳俱虚的，应阴阳双补。

中药的性味功能，也可用阴阳学说来概括，并以此作为临床用药的依据。如寒、凉药属阴，温、热药属阳；味酸、苦、咸的中药属阴，辛、甘、淡的中药属阳；具有收敛、沉降作用的中药属阴，具有发散、升浮作用的中药属阳。中医治病，就是根据病情阴阳偏盛、偏衰的情况，确定治疗原则的。治疗原则一旦确定，就结合药物的阴阳属性和作用，来选择使用相应的药物，从而达到治疗目的。

Section 2

Theory of Five Elements

1. The Formation of the Theory of Five Elements

Although the Chinese theory of the five elements and Greek theory of the four elements are different in history of formation, yet both of them belong to the earliesta tomic theory inessence. At first, the Chinese only knew that the five kinds of substances (wood, fire, earth, metal and water) were indispensable things in the daily life of mankind. Subsequently they made a generalization and deduction of the respective properties of the five kinds of substances and their relationship, so as to explain the whole material world. According to the theory of the five elements, wood, fire, earth, metal and water are five basic substances that constitute the material world. These substances are not only of the relations with generation and restriction but set in a state of constant motion and change. That is why it is known as the theory of the five elements or the doctrine of five evolutive phases.

2. The Content of the Theory of Five Elements

1) Attribution of Thing in Light of the Theory of Five Elements

In light of the theory of five elements, TCM has made a comprehensive comparison and study of all kinds of things and phenomena in nature as well as in the viscera, bowels, tissues,

第二节　五行学说

1．五行学说的形成

中国的五行学说与希腊的四元说形成的历史虽然不同，但其本质都是最早的原子论。最初，人们只是认识到木、火、土、金、水五种物质是人类生活中不可缺少的东西；后来，人们把这五种物质的属性及其相互关系加以抽象推演，用来说明整个物质世界。五行学说认为，木、火、土、金、水是构成物质世界的五种基本物质；这五种物质之间，不仅具有相互资生、相互制约的关系，而且处于不断的运动变化之中，故被称之为“五行”学说。

2．五行学说的内容

1）事物的五行分类

中医学运用五行学说，将自然界的各种事物与现象，以及人

physiology and pathology of the human body, attributed them respectively to one of the five elements, i.e., wood, fire, earth, metal and water in accordance with their different properties, functions and forms, thus expounding the physiology, pathology of the human body and the correlation between man and his natural surroundings. The following is a table showing the classification of things according to the theory of the five elements.

The Classification of Things According to the Theory of the Five Elements

Human Body					
five elements	viscera	bowels	five sense organs	five tissues	emotional activity
wood	liver	gall bladder	eye	tendon	anger
fire	heart	small intestine	tongue	vessel	joy
earth	spleen	stomach	mouth	muscle	overthinking
metal	lung	large intestine	nose	skin & hair	grief
water	kidney	urinary bladder	ear	bone	fear

体的脏腑、组织、生理、病理，做了广泛的比较和研究，采用“取类比象”的方法，按照事物的不同性质、作用与形态，分别归属于木、火、土、金、水“五行”之中，借以阐明人体的生理、病理以及人与自然环境间的相互联系。现将事物的五行归类列表介绍如下：

五行归类表

五行	人体				
	脏	腑	五官	五体	情志
木	肝	胆	目	筋	怒
火	心	小肠	舌	脉	喜
土	脾	胃	口	肉	思
金	肺	大肠	鼻	皮毛	悲
水	肾	膀胱	耳	骨	恐

Nature						
five elements	season	environ-mental factor	growth & development	colour	taste	orienta-tion
wood	spring	wind	germination	blue	sour	east
fire	summer	heat	growth	red	bitter	south
earth	late summer	dampness	transfor-mation	yellow	sweet	middle
metal	autumn	dryness	reaping	white	pungent	west
water	winter	cold	storing	black	salty	north

2) Generation, Restriction, Subjugation and Reverse Restriction among the Five Elements

Among the five elements, there exist the relations of generation, restriction, subjugation and reverse restriction.

Generation implies production and promotion. The order of generation is as follows: wood generates fire, fire generates earth, earth generates metal, metal generates water, and water, in its turn, generates wood. As far as the relationship of generation of each of the five elements is concerned, it is composed of two aspects — generating and being generated. The element that generates is called the mother, while the element that is generated is called the son. Hence, the relation of generating and being generated among the five elements is also known as that of mother and son. Take wood for example. Because wood produces fire, it is called the mother of fire. On the other hand it is produced by water, so it is called the son of water.

自然界						
五行	季节	气候	生长发育	颜色	五味	方位
木	春	风	生	青	酸	东
火	夏	热	长	赤	苦	南
土	长夏	湿	化	黄	甘	中
金	秋	燥	收	白	辛	西
水	冬	寒	藏	黑	咸	北

2)五行的生克乘侮

五行间存在着生、克、乘、侮的关系。

相生，含有相互资生和助长的意思。相生的次序是：木生火，火生土，土生金，金生水，水生木。在五行的相生关系中，任何一行都有"生我"、"我生"两方面的关系。生我者为母，我生者为子。所以五行的相生关系也称为母子关系。以木为例，由于木生火，故木为火之母；而木由水所生，故木又为水之子。

Restriction connotes bringing under control or restraint. So far as the relationship of restriction that the five elements possess is concerned, it works in the following order: wood restricts earth, earth water, water fire, fire metal, and metal wood. Each of the five elements has the chance of restricting and being restricted. Take wood for example. The element restricting wood is metal, and the element that is restricted by wood is earth.

In view of the correlations among things, neither generation nor restriction is dispensable. Without generation, there would be no birth and development; without restriction, excessive growth would result in harm. For instance, on one hand, wood generates fire, and on the other, it restricts earth; while earth, in its turn, generates metal and restricts water. Thus in generation there resides restriction, and in restriction there exists generation. They oppose each other and at the same time cooperate with each other, thus a relative balance is maintained between generation and restriction, and the normal growth and development of things is ensured.

Should one of the five elements be excessive or insufficient, there would appear the phenomena of abnormal restrictions, known as subjugation and reverse restriction.

By subjugation is meant that one element subdues the other when the latter is weak. It is the manifestation of abnormal coordination among things. For instance, if wood is in excess and metal can not exercise normal restriction on it, then the excessive wood will subjugate earth in such a way that earth will become weaker.

Reverse restriction means preying upon others. That is, when any one of the five elements is in excess, the one originally restricting it will be restricted by it instead. That is why we call it reverse restriction. For instance, the normal order of restriction is that metal restricts wood; but if wood is in excess or metal is insufficient, wood will restricts metal in the re-

相克有相互克制和约束的含义。五行的相克次序是：木克土，土克水，水克火，火克金，金克木。其中任何一行，都有“克我”、“我克”两方面的关系。以木为例，克木者为金，木克者为土。

在事物的相互关系中，不可无生，也不可无制，无生则不能发生、发展，无制则亢而为害。例如，木能生火，也能克土；土能生金，又能克水。这样，生中寓制，制中寓生，相反相成，并保持生克相对平衡，才能保证事物的正常发生与发展。

如果五行发生太过或不及，就会出现五行相互克伐的异常现象，称为“相乘”和“相侮”。

相乘，含有乘虚侵袭的意思，是事物间的关系失却正常协调的一种表现。如木气偏亢，而金又不能对木正常克制时，太过的木便去乘土，使土更虚。

相侮，含有恃强欺侮的意思。即五行中某一行本身太过，使原来克它的一行，不仅不能去制约它，反而被它所克制，故又称“反克”。例如：正常的相克关系是金克木，若木气偏亢，或金气不足，木就会反过来侮金。十分清楚，五行相

verse direction. It is clear that the order of reverse restriction is just opposite to that of restriction and that reverse restriction is undoubtedly a harmful one.

3. The Application of the Theory of Five Elements in TCM

In the science of TCM, the theory of five elements is used, in the main, to explain the physiology and pathology of the human body and to guide the clinical diagnosis and treatment.

1) Explaining the Correlations between the Five Viscera

The generation of the five elements can be used to expound the interdepending relations between the five viscera. For instance, the vital essence of the kidney (water) nourishes the liver (wood), which is known as water generating wood. The liver (wood) stores blood to nourish the heart (fire), which is termed wood generating fire. The heat of the heart (fire) warms the spleen (earth), which is called fire generating earth. The spleen (earth) transforms and distributes food essence to replenish the lung (metal), which is referred to as earth generating metal. The lung (metal) dredges the water passages to help the kidney (water), which is taken as metal generating water.

The restriction of the five elements can be used to explain the inter-restraining relations between the five viscera. For instance, the lung (metal) disperses and descends so as to restrain the exuberance of the liver (wood), which is known as metal restricting wood. The liver (wood) that functions well smoothes and regulates the stagnation of the *qi* of the spleen (earth), which is called as wood restricting earth. The function of the spleen (earth) plays in transporting, distributing and transforming nutrients and promoting water metabolism and may prevent the overflow of the water of the kidney (water), which is referred to as earth restricting water. The ascending of the kidney (water) can prevent the heart (fire) from hyperac-

侮恰与五行相克的次序相反。当然，五行相侮是一种克伐侵害关系。

3．五行学说在中医学中的应用

中医学借助五行学说，主要是用来解释人体的生理、病理，并指导临床诊断与治疗。

1）说明五脏之间的相互关系

五行的"相生"可用来说明五脏之间的相互资生关系。如肾(水)之精以养肝(木)，为水生木；肝(木)藏血以济心(火)，为木生火；心(火)之热以温脾(土)，为火生土；脾(土)化生水谷精微以充肺(金)，为土生金；肺(金)通调水道以助肾(水)，为金生水。

五行的"相克"可用来说明五脏之间的相互制约关系。如肺(金)清肃下降可抑制肝(木)的上亢，为金克木；肝(木)的条达可疏泄脾(土)气的壅滞，为木克土；脾(土)的运化可以防止肾(水)的泛

tivity, which is explained as water restricting fire.

2) Expounding Pathological Influences between the Five Viscera

As is known, the theories of sudjugation, reverse restriction, "illness of mother-organ involving son-organ", and "illness of son-organ involving mother-organ" concerning the five elements may be used to expound the pathological influences between the five viscera. Take lung trouble for example. If it results from heart trouble, that is regarded as "fire subjugating metal". If it is caused by liver (wood) trouble, that is referred to as "wood reversely restricting metal". If it is led by spleen (earth) trouble, that is looked upon as "illness of mother-organ involving son-organ". And if it is due to kidney (watei) trouble, that is taken as "illness of son-organ involving mother-organ".

3) Diagnosing and Treating Diseases

Because, in accordance with the atribution of things to the five elements, the five viscera have specific connections with the five colors (blue, red, yellow, white and black,) the five voices (shouting, laughing, singing, crying and moaning), the five kinds of flavours (sour, bitter, sweet, acrid and salty) as well as the relevant pulse conditions, one, when diagnosing, should do like this: first, synthesize the materials obtained through the four methods of diagnosis (observation, listening and smelling, inquiring, pulse feeling and palpation), and then, deduce what the disease is according to the theory of five elements. For instance, a blue face, preference for food with sour flavour and bowstring pulse condition may indicate liver disease; a red face, bitter taste in the mouth and overflowing pulse condition may suggest the hyperactivity of heart fire; the patient whose *qi* of the spleen is deficient looks blue because of "wood having subjugated earth"; the patient who has heart trouble

滥，为土克水；肾(水)上承，可防止心(火)过于亢烈，为水克火。

2）说明五脏之间的病理影响

五行的“相乘”、“相侮”、“母病及子”、“子病及母”可用来说明脏腑间的病理影响。以肺病为例，如因心(火)病影响而致肺(金)病，为“火乘金”；如因肝(木)病影响而致肺(金)病，为“木侮金”；如因脾(土)病影响而致肺(金)病，为“母病及子”；如因肾(水)病影响而致肺(金)病，为“子病及母”。

3）用于诊断和治疗

由于五脏与五色、五音、五味及相关脉象在五行分类归属上有着特定的联系，故诊断时可综合四诊所得的材料，根据五行学说来推断病情。如面见青色，喜食酸食，脉见弦象，可诊为肝病；面见赤色，口味苦，脉象洪，可诊为心火亢盛；脾虚的病人，面

looks dark because of "water having restricted fire", to mention but a few.

In treatment, the theory of five elements, on the one hand, is used to prevent the transmission of diseases. As The 77th Problem, a chapter of ***Classic On Medical Problems***, says, "When liver disease occurs, it will spread to the spleen, so the *qi* of the spleen should be reinforced before it is affected." On the other hand, the theory of five elements may be used to help work out the principle and method of treatment. For instance, The 69th Problem, a chapter of ***Classic On Medical Problems***, points out that "if hypofunction is found in the son-organ, the mother-organ should be tonified; if hyperfunction is found in the mother-organ, the son-organ shonld be treated with purgation", to mention but a few. Physicians of later generations have applied the law of generation, restriction, subjugation and reverse restriction of the five elements to work out many effective and specific treating methods such as reinforcing earth to generate metal (strengthening the function of the spleen to benefit the lung), replenishing water to nourish wood (nourishing the essence of the kidney to benefit the liver), supporting earth to restrict wood (supplementing the function of the spleen to treat hyperactivity of the liver), and strengthening water to control fire (replenishing the essence of the kidney to treat hyperactivity of the heart), and so on

In the science of acupuncture and moxibustion, the five kinds of points of the 12 channels distributed at the ends of the extremities, i.e., the *Jing* (well) Points, the *Ying* (spring) Points, the *Shu* (stream) Points, the *Jing* (river) Points and the *He* (sea) Points, are respectively included in the five elements — wood, fire, earth, metal and water. In clinical treatment, these points may be chosen according to the specific state of certain illness that is being treated and in accordance with the law of generation, restriction, subjugation and reverse resrtiction of the five elements.

见青色，为木乘土；心脏病人，面见黑色，为水克火等。

五行学说用于治疗，一是控制疾病的传变，如《难经·七十七难》"见肝之病，则知肝当传之于脾，故先当实其脾气"；二是帮助制定治疗原则与方法，如《难经·六十九难》："虚则补其母，实则泻其子"等。后世医家运用五行的规律，制定了许多行之有效的治疗方法，如培土生金、滋水涵木、扶土抑木和壮水制火等。

针灸学将十二经脉分布在四肢末端的井、荥、俞、经、合五种穴位分属于木、火、土、金、水。临床可根据具体病情，运用五行的生克乘侮规律进行选穴治疗。

From above, it has been known that the theory of *yin* and *yang* is used to state the two components of one thing, or the relations of opposition, interdependence, waxing and waning, and the transformation between two opposite things; while the theory of five elements is used mainly to exlpain the property and correlation among things according to the attribution of things to the five elements as well as the law of generation, restriction, subjugation and reverse restriction of the five elements. But do remember that both theories are often combined when used.

由上可知，阴阳学说主要是说明同一事物的两个方面，或两个相对事物的对立、互根、消长、转化关系；五行学说则主要是以事物属性的五行归类及其生克乘侮，来说明事物的性质及其相互关系。但在中医理论中，二者多互相联系，结合运用。

Chapter Three

The Theory of Viscera and Bowels

In TCM, the internal organs of the human body are divided into three groups: "five viscera", "six bowels" and "extraordinary organs". The five viscera include the heart, the liver, the spleen the lung and the kidney. Preserving vital substances is their common characteristic. The six bowels contain the gallbladder, the stomach, the large intestine, the small intestine, the urinary bladder and the triple warmer. Their common characteristic is transmitting and digesting water and food. The extraordinary organs refer to the brain, the medulla, the bone, the blood vessel, the gallbladder and the woman's uterus — six organs or tissues in all. "*Qi*" — the sound of a Chinese character — means "extra", while "*heng*" — the sound of another Chinese character — means "ordinary". Although they may also be called "bowels", their functions are different from those of "the six bowels" mentioned above. So they are named "extraordinary organs".

The theory of viscera and bowels is one concerning the studies of the physiological functions and pathological changes of every organ of the human body, and their interrelationships. The formation of this theory is closely related to the following three factors, the first is ancient anatomical knowledge. For instance, *Jingshui Pian*", a chapter on the fluid in the channels in the book ***Miraculous Pivot***, says: "When an eight-*chi*-tall adult stands upright before you, yocu can take his full height. When he dies, you can observe the details of his body through an autopsy. So you can get a general idea of whether his internal organs are solid or fragile, whether his bowels are large or small, whether there is a lot or a little food within his stomach, and whether his blood vessels are long or short, and so on and so forth."

第 三 章

脏腑学说

中医将人体的内脏分成五脏、六腑和奇恒之腑三类。五脏，即心、肝、脾、肺、肾，它们的共同特点是具有贮藏精气的功能。六腑，即胆、胃、大肠、小肠、膀胱、三焦，它们的共同特点是具有传送、消化水谷的功能。奇恒之腑包括脑、髓、骨、脉、胆、女子胞六种器官、组织。奇者，异也；恒者，常者。它们虽名曰腑，但其功能与腑有别，故名“奇恒之腑”。

脏腑学说，是研究人体各脏腑的生理功能、病理变化及其相互关系的学说。这一学说的形成，主要有三个方面：一是古代的解剖知识，如《灵枢·经水篇》说：“夫八尺之士，皮肉在此，外可度量切循而得之。其死可解剖而视之。其脏之坚脆，腑之大小，谷之多少，脉之长短，……皆有大数。”可见早在2,000多年前中医

This shows that as early as 2,000 years before TCM had already begun to perform autopsies on human. The second factor is the observation of physiological and pathological phenomena. For example, if one catches cold because his skin has been affected by cold, he will have the signs and symptoms of a disorder of the respiratory system such as nasal obstruction, rhinorrhea and cough. That is why TCM believes that the skin and hair have something to do with the nose and lung, that is to say, with the respiratory system. The third factor is the summarization of long-term medical experiences. For instance, quite a few medicines which have the function of reinforcing the vital energy or essence of the kidney can accelerate the healing of the bone. This brings about the saying that the condition of the kidney determines the condition of the bone.

It is needed to point out especially that TCM's names of the internal organs of the human body are basically the same as those used in Western medicine, but all concepts are not the same. For example, the functions of an organ in TCM may contain the functions of many organs in Western medicine. Meanwhile, the function of an organ in Western medicine may be contained in the functions of several viscera and bowels in TCM. This is because TCM's viscus or bowel is not only an anatomic unit, but also a concept of physiology and pathology, and the latter is more important. For instance, the heart in TCM does refer to the same anatomic entity as in Western medicine. In addition, however, it also refers to some of the functions of the nervous system, especially some of those of the brain. The difference in concepts between TCM and Western medicine is mainly due to the difference in the way of seeing things. TCM gathers its knowledge of the internal organs mainly from repeated practice and observation, whereas Western medicine bases its knowledge mainly on repeated autopsies, experiments and summarizations. Hence, in learning the theory of TCM concerning viscera and bowels, you should, first of

就已开始对人体进行解剖。二是对生理、病理现象的观察，如皮肤受凉而感冒，可出现鼻塞、流涕、咳嗽等肺系症状，因而认为皮毛与鼻、肺(呼吸系)有联系；三是长期医疗经验的总结，如不少补肾药能加速骨折的愈合，因而产生了"肾主骨"之说。

需要特别指出的是，中医的脏器名称虽与西医基本相同，但其概念并不完全一致。中医某一脏器的功能可以包含西医数个脏器的功能；而西医某一脏器的功能，又可能分散在中医的好几个脏腑之中。这是因为中医的脏和腑，不单纯是一个解剖学单位，更重要的是一个生理、病理学概念。例如：中医的心，除代表西医解剖学上的实体"心脏"外，还包括神经系统，特别是大脑的某些功能。中西医在概念上的这一差异主要是由于二者在认识方法上的不同所造成的。如前所述，中医对脏腑的认识主要是通过反复的实践、观察、抽象而来；而西医对脏器的认识则主要以反复的解剖、实验、总结为依据。因此，我们在学习时应首先搞清中

all, have a clear idea of what it is all about, and then make further inquiries and studies of it through the step-by-step adoption of modern technical know-how and method so as to bring to light its essence.

Section 1

Five Viscera (*Zang*-organ)

1. The Heart (and the Pericardium)

The heart lies in the chest and takes a position left of the centre. TCM believes that it is the most important organ of the human body and governs all the viscera and bowels. The book, ***Canon of Medicine*** says, "The heart is the monarch of all the organs". Moreover, TCM divides the heart itself into the *yin* (vital essence) of the heart and the *yang* (vital function) of the heart. The former refers to the material structures, including the blood of the heart. The latter refers to its function and heat, including the *qi* (functional activities). The blood of the heart means the blood controlled by the heart. The *qi* of the heart means the function of the heart. According to TCM, the main physiological functions of the heart are as follows:

1) Controlling Blood Circulation

By blood circulation, we suggest both blood and its vessels. Blood vessels are the ducts through which blood flows and blood is the content of the blood vessels. The heart is linked with the blood vessels to form a closed system. The heart is beating continuously to propel the blood to flow and circulate within the blood vessels throughout the body. TCM believes that the *qi* of the heart is the driving force of the heart's beating. Only when the *qi* of the heart is sufficient, can the heart keep normal strength, rate and rhythm. Whether the *qi* of the heart is

医脏腑学说的本来含义，然后再逐步采用现代科学的知识和方法进一步探讨、研究，以揭示其实质。

第一节　五　脏

1. 心(附心包)

心位于胸中偏左。中医认为它是人体最重要的脏器，其他脏腑都是在心的统一支配下进行活动，所以《内经》称之为“君主之官”。中医将心脏本身又分为心阴，即心的物质结构，亦包括心血；心阳，即心的功能与热力，亦包括心气；心血，即心所主的血液；心气，即心的功能。中医认为，心的主要生理功能如下：

1) 主血脉

血脉包括血液和脉管。脉管是血液运行的通道，血是脉管的内容物。心与脉管相通，构成了一个密闭的系统。心脏不停地搏动，推动着血液在全身脉管中流动、循环。中医认为，心气是心

sufficient or not and whether the blood of the heart is sufficient or not may both be shown from the condition of the pulse. For instance, an empty pulse with little strength shows an insufficiency of the *qi* of the heart; a fine and weak pulse shows a deficiency of the blood of the heart; a rough and intermittent pulse shows stagnation of the blood of the heart, to mention but a few.

2) Taking Charge of Mental Activities

TCM believes all the higher nervous activities such as mental, conscious and thinking ones, rseult mainly from the functions of the heart. If one's heart functions normally in controlling mental activities, one will be full of vigour, and have healthy consciousness and sound mental activities. But when there is something wrong with this function, then abnormalities will be seen, such as insanity from mental disturbance due to phlegmatic fire, and palpitation, insomnia and dream-disturbed sleep due to an insufficiency of the blood of the heart. The treatment of these abnormalities is always based on an overall analysis of the heart condition.

3) Sweat as the Fluid of the Heart

Sweat comes from body fluid. Body fluid is the most important component of the blood. Blood circulation is controlled by the heart. So it can be said: "Blood and sweat have the same source" and "Sweat is the fluid of the heart". TCM believes that too much perspiration suggests easy consumption of the blood and *qi* of the heart, resulting in palpitation and continuous violent beating of the heart. Furthermore,profuse sweating will damage the *yang* of the heart, resulting in a dangerously excessive loss of the fluid. It is easy for those who suffer from a deficiency of the *yang* of the heart to perspire spontaneously, and for those whose *yin* of the heart is insufficient to sweat at night.

脏搏动的动力。心气充足，才能维持正常的心力、心率和心律。心气的强弱、心血的盛衰，都可从脉搏反映出来。例如：心气不足则脉虚无力；心血不足则脉细而弱；心血瘀阻则脉涩结代。

2）主神志

凡精神、意识、思维等高级神经的活动，中医认为主要是心的功能。如果心主神志的功能正常，则人的精神充沛，意识清楚，思维智敏；如发生障碍，则出现神志方面的异常，如痰火扰心的癫狂，心血不足的失眠、多梦、心悸等。治疗时都是从心论治。

3）汗为心之液

由于汗为津液所化生，津液是血液的重要组成部分，心主血脉，故有“血汗同源”、“汗为心之液”的说法。中医认为，汗出过多，易耗伤心血、心气，出现心悸、怔忡等；大汗淋漓则可进一步损及心阳，出现“大汗亡阳”的危象；心阳虚者易自汗；心阴虚者易盗汗。

4) Having Relations with the Tongue and Face

TCM believes, "The heart has its specific opening in the tongue proper"; "The tongue is the sprout of the heart"; "The reticular branch conduits of the heart channels ascend and connect with the tongue"; "The heart has its outward manifestation in the face or complexion". The face is rich in blood vessels, and its colour can show how the heart functions. Therefore, in TCM, the conditions of the heart and the blood are often learned by observing the tongue and face. For instance, when the heart functions well and when the blood is plentiful, the face will be red and bright, and so will be the tongue. When the blood of the heart is insufficient, the face will be pale, the tongue will be pale and white. When there is a stagnation of the blood of the heart, the face will be cyanosed, the tongue dark purple or with petechiae and ecchymoses. When the heart does not function normally in controlling mental activities, tongue rigidity, delirium or aphasia will occur.

Also the nourishment of the hair comes from the blood. That is why it is said that hair is the surplus of the blood. So, when the blood of the heart is insufficient, the hair will be withered.

Supplement: Pericardium

Pericardium is the peripheral tissue of the heart, which plays the part of protection. External pathogenic factors often invade the pericardium before they attack the heart. For instance, in TCM, the high fever, coma and red tongue occurring in the course of a febrile disease are often described as "the attack of the pericardium by pathogenic heat". In fact the signs and symptoms occurring after the pericardium has been invaded by external pathogenic factors are the same as those appearing after the heart has been attacked.

Note: From the physiology and pathology of the heart

4)心与舌、面的联系

中医认为，“心开窍与舌”，“舌为心之苗”，“心经的别络上系于舌”；“其华在面”，即面部血管丰富，面部色泽能反映心的功能状态。因此，中医常通过察舌和面来测知心与血的情况。例如：心功能良好，血液充盈，则面部红润光泽，舌质红活；心血不足，则面色苍白，舌质淡白；心血瘀阻，则面色青紫，舌质紫暗，或有瘀点、瘀斑；心主神志的功能异常，则见舌强、语謇或失语等。

此外，毛发的营养来源于血，故有“发为血之余”的说法。若心血不足、可出现毛发枯槁等。

附：心包

心包是心脏的外围组织，有保护心脏的作用。外邪犯心，常先侵犯心包。例如：热病过程中如出现高热、神昏、舌质红降等，中医称之为“热入心包”。实际上，心包受邪后所出现的病症与心是一致的。

stated above, it is easy to see that the term "heart" in TCM basically suggests all the functions of the heart and the part of the functions of the nervous system in Western medicine.

2. The Lung

The lung consisting of the two lobes is located in the chest, one on the left, the other on the right. It is connected with larynx through the bronchioles, bronchi and trachea, and has its opening in the nose. TCM usually divides the lung into the *yin* of the lung, i.e., the material structures of the lung, and the *qi* of the lung, i.e., the physiological functions of the lung. In TCM literature, the terms "the *yang* of the lung" and "the blood of the lung" are rarely used. The main physiological functions of the lung are as follows:

1) Taking Charge of *Qi*

The lung taking charge of *qi* means that the lung has the function to control the *qi* of the human body. This function is shown in two ways — taking charge of the *qi* of respiration and operating the *qi* of the whole body.

(1) Taking Charge of the *Qi* of Respiration

The lung performs the function of respiration. It is the chief organ for exchanging air between the interior and the exterior of the body. The human body takes in fresh air (oxygen) and expels waste gas (carbon dioxide) by the respiratory function of the lung, and in so doing keep the metabolism of the human body functioning smoothly. If the lung's functions are abnormal due to being harmed by external pathogenic factors, such signs and symptoms due to the disorders of the respiratory system as cough, asthmatic breathing and difficulty in breathing will occur.

(2) Operating the *Qi* of the Whole Body

That the lung operates the *qi* of the whole body can be

按语：从上述的生理、病理来看，中医的"心"基本包括西医的心脏以及部分神经系统的功能。

2、肺

肺位于胸中，左右各一，上通气管、喉咙，开窍于鼻。中医习惯将肺本身又分为肺阴，即肺的物质结构；肺气，即肺的生理功能。而在中医文献中，称肺阳、肺血者较少。肺的主要生理功能如下：

1)肺主气

肺主气是指肺有主持人体之气的功能，这包括两个方面，即主呼吸之气和主一身之气。

(1)主呼吸之气

肺有主司呼吸的作用，为体内外气体交换的主要器官。人体通过肺的呼吸功能，吸入自然界的清气(氧气)，呼出体内的浊气(二氧化碳)，从而保证人体新陈代谢的正常进行。如果肺受邪而功能异常，可出现咳嗽、气喘、呼吸不利等呼吸系症状。

(2)主一身之气

这体现在两个方面：一是肺与"宗气"的生成有关。"宗气"是

seen in two aspects:

The first is that the lung takes part in the forming of "*zong qi*" (pectoral energy). Fresh air inhaled by the lung (cosmic energy) and food essence mix and accumulate in the chest to form *zong qi*. *Zong qi* exits from the larynx, thus promoting the lung's respiratory activities. It spreads to all parts of the body by way of the heart channels, thus warming the viscera, bowels and tissues, and maintaining normal physiological activities.

The second is that the lung has the function of operating and regulating the *qi* of the whole body to ascend or descend, enter or exit. If this function of the lung is abnormal, the formation of *zong qi*, and the ascending or descending and entering or exiting out of the mechanism of the *qi* of the whole body will be affected, manifested as shortness of breath, low voice, tiredness, lassitude and so on.

2) Activating the Flow of *Qi*, Food Essence and Body Fluid, Clearing the Inspired Air and Keeping It Flowing Downward and Helping Maintain Normal Water Metabolism

By activating the flow of *qi*, food essence and body fluid we mean the lung has the function of disseminating defending *qi*, food essence and body fluid throughout the body so as to nourish the body and to warm and moisten the muscles, skin and hair. The book ***Classic of Acupuncture*** says, "If the upper warmer (upper portion of the body cavity) functions well, it can activate the flow of *qi*, food essence and body fluid, nourish the skin and the whole body, moisten and brighten the hair, as the rain and dew moisten young crops." Here, "the upper warmer's functioning well" means the lung's function of activating the flow of *qi*, food essence and body fluid.

Cleaning the inspired air and keeping it flowing downward

由肺吸入的清气与水谷之精气结合，积于胸中而成。宗气上出喉咙，能促进肺的呼吸运动；通过心脉而布散全身，以温煦各脏腑、组织，并维持其正常生理活动。二是肺有主持、调节全身气机升降出入的作用。因此，肺主一身之气的功能异常，可影响宗气的生成和全身气机的升降出入运动，表现为气短、声低、体倦、乏力等。

2)主宣发、肃降、行水

肺主宣发，是指肺有将卫气、水谷精微输布全身，以充养身体，温润肌腠、皮毛的作用。《针经》说："上焦开发，宣五谷味，熏肤、充身、泽毛，若雾露之溉，是谓气。"这里所说的"上焦开发"，主要是指肺的宣发功能。

肃降，即清肃下降的意思。肺居胸中，位于上焦，其气以清

mean clarifying and sending down the *qi* of the lung. As the lung is within the chest, lying in the upper warmer, it is normal for its *qi* to descend. If the lung's *qi* fails to descend, cough, asthmatic breathing, stuffy sensation in the chest and the like will appear. In addition, this lung's function of descending is associated with the metabolism of water. That is, it can cause water in the upper warmer to descend into the kidney and urinary bladder, thus keeping urination smooth and the metabolism of water normal. This is the reason for the sayings: "The lung helps maintain normal water metabolism." and "The lung has the function of dredging water passages." If there is something wrong with this function of the lung, the dissemination and discharge of water will be disturbed, which results in dysuria, edema and phlegm-retention diseases.

The lung's two functions of dispersing and descending are two components which oppose and yet complement each other. Without normal dispersing, there will not be good descending and vice versa. The coordination of dispersing and descending keeps breathing even and the *qi* of the lung passing in and out smoothly. If they are not coordinated, pathological changes such as "disturbance of the *qi* of the lung" and "impairment of the normal function of clarifying and sending down the *qi* of the lung" will appear. The clinical manifestations of these are cough, asthmatic breathing ,stuffiness in the chest, hypochondriac distention and so on.

3) Being Associated with the Skin and Hair and Having Its Special Opening in the Nose

When we talk about the skin and hair, we have in our minds the skin surface, sweat glands, hair and other relevant tissues. Being associated with the skin and hair means that the lung has the function of disseminating body fluid and activating defending energy to the skin and hair so that the skin surface can be made moist and bright, the skin and muscles compact and the

肃下降为顺。肺失肃降，可出现咳逆、喘息、胸闷等。此外，肺的肃降还与水液代谢有关。通过这一功能，可使上焦水液不断地下输肾与膀胱，从而保持小便通利，水液代谢正常，故有“肺主行水”、“通调水道”的说法。如肺的这一功能异常，则水的输布、排泄障碍，出现小便不利、水肿和痰饮等。

肺的宣布与肃降，是相辅相成的两个方面。没有正常的宣发，就不能很好地肃降；没有正常的肃降，也就不能很好地宣发。宣发与肃降协调，则肺气出入通畅，呼吸调匀。如果二者失调，就会出现“肺气不宣”或“肺失肃降”的病变，表现为咳嗽、喘息、胸闷、胁胀等。

3)肺合皮毛，开窍于鼻

皮毛，包括皮肤、汗腺、毛发等组织。肺合皮毛，是说肺能输布津液、宣发卫气于皮毛，使皮肤润泽，肌腠致密，抵御外邪

ability to fight against external pathogenic factors can be enhanced. A deficiency of the *qi* of the lung brings on an unconsolidated defending energy whose manifestations are sweating spontaneously as well as being susceptible to the common cold due to a disability in fighting against external pathogenic factors.

The nose is the doorway of the lung through which the air enters and exits. Its functions of ventilation and smelling are mainly dependent on the action of the *qi* of the lung. The free movement of the *qi* of the lung keeps respiration unobstructed and gives a keen sense of smell. Invasion of the lung by external pathogenic factors blocks the movement of the *qi* of the lung, which results in nasal obstruction, watery nasal discharge and a hyposmia. The invasion of the lung by pathogenic heat factor often has the sign of "the wings of the nose flapping". The nose is the passage through which pathogens invade the lung, because it is the opening of the lung. This is why epidemic febrile pathogenic factors always attack the lung by way of the nose.

4) Being a Delicate Organ Leading up to the Larynx

In fact the lung is directly exposed to external air. As a result it is open to attack from every kind of external pathogenic factor. Therefore there is a saying: "The lung is a delicate organ, vulnerable to the attack of external influences."

The larynx is not only a part of the respiratory tract but also the phonetic organ, through which the lung channels pass. So its ventilation and phonation directly relate to the lung. A sufficiency of the *qi* of the lung produces a loud voice; while a deficiency makes the voice low. Also, a deficiency of the *yin* of the lung may lead to a hoarse voice and even aphonia.

Note: From what has been said above about the physiology and pathology of the lung, it can be seen that the lung, in TCM, basically plays the same part as the respiratory system in Western medicine, and are related to water metabolism, blood circulation and the functions of the vegetative nervous system and the immune system.

的能力增强。肺气虚则体表不固，常自汗出；卫气不固则抵御外邪的能力降低，而易于感冒。

鼻是肺的门户，为气体出入的通道，其通气和嗅觉功能，主要依赖肺气的作用。肺气通利，则呼吸通畅，嗅觉灵敏；外邪犯肺，肺气不利，则见鼻塞、流涕、嗅觉不灵；邪热壅肺，则常出现鼻翼煽动。正由于鼻为肺窍，故鼻又常成为邪气侵犯肺脏的通道，温邪犯肺，多由口鼻而入。

4）肺为娇脏，上连于喉

肺与外界空气直接接触，故各种外邪易侵犯肺脏而发病，因而有“肺为娇脏”的说法。

喉不仅是呼吸的通道，而且也是发音的器官，肺的经脉从这里通过，故喉的通气、发音直接与肺有关。如肺气足则声音洪亮，肺气虚常声音低微；肺阴虚还可引起声音嘶哑、失音等。

按语：从上述肺的生理、病理看来，中医的肺基本概括了西医呼吸系统的功能，并与水液代谢、血液循环、植物神经以及免疫系统的功能有关。

3. The Spleen

TCM is world apart from Western medicine in terms of understanding the spleen. TCM believes that the spleen lies in the middle warmer (the middle portion of the body cavity) and is the main organ of the digestive system. Not only that, it divides the spleen into the *yin* of the spleen (its material structures) and the *yang* of the spleen (its functions and heat). The *qi* of the spleen simply refers to its functions. In TCM literature, the term "the blood of the spleen" is uncommon. The main functions of the spleen are as follows:

1) Transporting, Distributing and Transforming Nutrients

(1) Transporting, Distributing and Transforming Water and Food

TCM believes that the food taken into the stomach is digested both by the stomach and the spleen, and then, through the pylorus, sent downwards into the small intestine to undergo the process of "differentiating pure substance from turbid substance". The pure part (food essence) is absorbed by the spleen and transported to all parts of the body so that the five viscera, six bowels, limbs, bones, hair and tendons are nourished. TCM says: "The spleen provides the material basis for the acquired constitution" and "The spleen is the source of producing the *qi* and blood." Why ? Because water and food are not only the chief source of the nutrients which man needs to keep his life activites after birth, but also the material basis for producing *qi* and blood, and, what is more, it is the spleen that transports, distributes and transforms nutrients. A dysfunction of the spleen in transporting, distributing and transforming nutrients will cause poor appetite, indigestion, fullness and distension in the epigastrium, loose stools, lassitude, loss of weight and other diseases due to the deficiency of both *qi* and blood.

(2) Promoting Water Metabolism

3. 脾

中医对脾的认识与西医相差甚远，认为它位于中焦，是消化系统的主要脏器，并将脾本身又分为脾阴，即脾的物质、结构；脾阳，即脾的功能与热力；脾气，即脾的功能。在中医文献中，单称“脾血”者少。脾的主要功能如下：

1）主运化

（1）运化水谷

中医认为，饮食入胃，须经过胃与脾的共同消化，然后通过幽门下送小肠进行“泌别清浊”。其“清”的部分（即水谷之精微）再由脾吸收并输送到全身，以营养五脏六腑、四肢百骸以及皮毛、筋骨等组织、器官。由于饮食水谷是人出生之后维持生命活动所需营养物质的主要来源，也是生成气血的物质基础，而饮食水谷的运化又由脾所主，所以有“脾为后天之本”、“气血生化之源”的说法。如脾运化水谷的功能异常，就会出现食欲不振、消化不良腹胀、便溏、倦怠、消瘦和气血虚弱的病症。

（2）运化水湿

The spleen helps in absorbing and transporting water. The abnormality of this function will induce every kind of disease resulting from the retention of water, e.g. edema, damp-phlegm, diarrhea, etc.

The spleen's function of promoting water metabolism takes place at the same time as that of transporting, distributing and transforming nutrients. These two functions are associated with, and influence, each other. A disorder in either one will induce an abnormality in the other. Therefore, one is often followed by the other in pathology. In treating either of them, the method of invigorating the spleen should be used.

2) Keeping Blood Circulating within the Vessels

The spleen has the function of controlling all the blood of the body and keeping it circulating normally within the vessels. If it loses this function because of a deficiency of its *qi*, the blood will not flow normally within the vessels but will extravasate from them. In this case, besides some signs and symptoms due to a deficiency of the *qi* of the spleen, certain kinds of chronic hemorrhages such as blood in the stool, purpura, uterine bleeding and others will occur. In treating these disorders, the spleen should be invigorated, the *qi* should be replensihed and bleeding should be controlled.

3) Having Relationship with the Muscles, Limbs and Lips

The spleen has the function of nourishing the muscles and limbs. When the spleen functions well in transportation, distribution and transformation, the food essence is distributed throughout the body so that the muscles are well-developed and strong and the limbs have strength to move, because they receive plentiful nutrients. If the spleen does not function well,the muscles will be thin, the limbs will be slack or too weak to function, because they can not receive enough nutrients.

脾参与水液的吸收和转输。若这一功能失常，可引起水液潴留致成的各种病症，如水肿、痰湿、泄泻等。

脾运化水谷和运化水湿的功能是同时进行，并相互联系、相互影响的。某一种功能障碍，常可导致另一种功能异常，故二者在病理上常常互见，治疗均需用健脾法。

2）主统血

是指脾气有统摄全身血液使之在脉管中正常运行而不致溢出脉外的功能。如脾气虚弱失去统血的功能，则“血不循经”，溢于脉外，除出现一些脾气虚的症状外，同时还出现某种出血证，如便血、皮下出血、子宫出血等，治疗则采用健脾、益气、摄血法。

3）脾与肌肉、四肢、口唇的关系

脾主肌肉、四肢，脾气健运，精微四布，营养充足，则肌肉丰满壮实，四肢活动有力。若脾失健运，营养不足，则出现肌肉瘦削、四肢倦怠无力或痿弱不用。

"The spleen has its 'special body opening' in the mouth." "It has its outward manifestations in the lips." The strong and vigorous *qi* of the spleen results in good appetite, normal taste, red and bright lips. A dysfunction of the spleen in transporting, distributing and transforming nutrients leads to poor appetite, ineffective taste and pale or yellowish whithered lips. A disturbance of the spleen by pathogenic damp factors also results in a sticky, sweet taste in the mouth, and should be treated with drugs, such as eupatorium (*Herba Eupatorii*), which resolve dampness and enliven the spleen.

In addition to what has been said above, the tendency of *qi* of the spleen is ascending. It has the function of sending food essence upward to the lung and fixing internal organs at their original locations. If the *qi* of the spleen does not go upward but downward (which is called, in TCM, the sinking of the *qi* of the middle warmer), permanent diarrhea, prolapse of the rectum and uterus and ptosis of other internal organs will occur. In treating these, the decoction of reinforcing the middle warmer and replenishing the *qi* is often prescribed. The spleen also has the physiological characteristic of liking dryness but hating dampness. Therefore, a dysfunction of the spleen in transportation and transformation due to a deficiency of the *qi* of the spleen is most liable to produce dampness, while excessive dampness will most likely disturb the spleen.

Note: From the physiology and pathology of the spleen stated above, it can be seen that the theory of spleen in TCM is concerned with most of the functions of the digestive system that Western medicine deals with, but is also related to blood coagulation and body fluid metabolism.

Finally, it is needed to point out that in TCM literature, the pancreas has not been mentioned. Some scholars believe that the spleen in TCM includes the pancreas.

“脾开窍于口”，“其华在唇”。脾气健旺，则食欲旺盛，口味正常，口唇红润光泽。脾失健运，则食欲不振，口中乏味，口唇色淡或萎黄不泽。湿邪困脾，还可引起口腻、口甜，治疗习惯采用化湿醒脾药，如佩兰等。

此外，脾气宜升，有升清、固摄的作用。所谓“升清”，是指精微物质的上升与输布；所谓“固摄”，是指保持内脏固定在正常位置而不垂。如脾气不升反而下陷（中医称为“中气下陷”），可出现久泻、脱肛、子宫下垂以及其他内脏下垂。治疗多用补中益气汤。脾还有喜燥恶湿的生理特性，故脾虚不运，最易生湿；而湿邪过盛，又最易困脾。

按语：从上述脾的生理、病理来看，中医的脾包含了西医之消化系统的大部分功能，并与血液凝固、体液代谢等有关。

此外，在中医文献中，尚无“胰腺”这一脏器。有的学者认为，中医的脾亦包括“胰腺”在内。

4. The Liver

The liver lies in the upper part of the abdomen on the right side, under the diaphragm, slightly to the right inside cf the right ribs. Its channels are distributed throughout the right and left ribs. TCM differentiates the liver as the *yin* of the liver (its material structures, including the blood stored in it) and the *yang* of the liver (its functions and heat, including the *qi* of the liver — its functions). The chief physiological functions of the liver are as follows:

1) Smoothing and Regulating the Flow of Vital Energy and Blood

Ancient medical men believed that a wood or a tree tended to spread out freely, so did the liver corresponding to this element. This is why the liver is classified as "wood" in the five elements. The liver's function in promoting unrestrained and free movement of *qi* is shown in the following three aspects:

(1) Regulating Mind and Mood

TCM believes that the mental activities of human beings are controlled by the heart and have something to do with the liver's function of smoothing and regulating the flow of vital energy and blood. When this function of the liver is normal the human body will coordinate its mental and moral activities well, which is indicated by happiness, being at ease, being able to reason and sensitivity. But when the liver does not perform this function well, the human body will fail to coordinate its mental and moral activities. This is indicated by dullness, anxiety, depression, belching, sighing, distension and stuffy sensation in the breast and hypochondria. When the liver performs this function to excess, excitatory state such as restlessness of the mind, irascibility, dizziness, a sensation of distension of the head, headache, insomnia and dream-distu rbed sleep may be present.

4. 肝

肝位于右上腹内，横膈下稍偏右，右肋之内。其经脉布两肋。中医将肝本身又分为肝阴，即肝的物质结构，包括肝血，即肝所藏的血液；肝阳，肝的功能与热力，包括肝气，即肝的功能。肝的主要生理功能如下：

1)主疏泄

古人以木气的冲和条达之象来形容肝的疏泄功能，故在五行中将其归属于木。其疏泄功能主要表现在以下三个方面：

(1)调节精神情志

中医认为，人的精神活动除由心所主外，还与肝的疏泄功能有关。肝的这一功能正常，人体就能较好地协调自身的精神、情志活动，表现为精神愉快、心情舒畅、理智灵敏；疏泄不及，则表现为精神抑郁、多愁善虑、沉闷欲哭、嗳气太息、胸胁胀闷等；疏泄太过，则表现为兴奋状态，如烦躁易怒、头晕胀痛、失眠多梦等。

(2) Promoting Digestion and Absorption

The liver's function of smoothing and regulating the flow of vital energy and blood helps the spleen in sending food essence and water up and the stomach in sending food contents down and secretion of bile, so that the function of digestion and absorption is kept normal. If this function of the liver does not work well, the ascending and descending *qi* of the spleen and stomach will be affected. The bile excretion will also be obstructed. This results in signs and symptoms of an abnormality in the digestive function, e.g., poor appetite, indigestion, belching, vomiting of sour fluid or distension of the abdomen, and diarrhea. TCM refers to this as "incoordination between the liver and the stomach or the spleen".

(3) Keeping *Qi* and Blood Moving Normally

The liver's function of smoothing and regulating the flow of vital energy and blood exerts a direct influence on the free movement of *qi*. The liver's dysfunction in promoting the free movement of *qi* causes the flow of *qi* to be obstructed, which is indicated by pain and distension in the hypochondria, the breasts and lower abdomen. *Qi* is the driving force in the circulation of blood. The flow of *qi* is followed by blood circulation. Blood stasis takes place after the stagnation of *qi*. The liver's dysfunction in promoting free movement of *qi* and blood stasis due to the stagnation of *qi* leads to pricking pain in the breast and hypochondria, even mass in the abdomen with fixed shape and localized pain, tumor, and possibly abnormal menstruation, dysmenorrhea and amenorrhea in women.

Furthermore, the liver's function of smoothing and regulating the flow of vital energy and blood also has the action of removing stagnant vital energy from the triple warmer as well as dregding the water passages. Also when the liver does not work well in promoting the free movement of *qi*, hydroperitoneum and edema may, sometimes, occur.

（2）促进消化吸收

肝的疏泄功能有助于脾胃的升降和胆汁的分泌，以保持正常的消化、吸收功能。如肝失疏泄，为影响脾胃之气的升降和胆汁的排泄，从而出现消化功能异常的症状，如食欲不振、消化不良、嗳气泛酸，或腹胀、腹泻等，中医称为“肝胃不和”或“肝脾不和”。

（3）维持气血运行

肝的疏泄功能直接影响着气机的调畅。如肝失疏泄，气机阻滞，可出现胸胁、两乳或少腹胀痛。气是血液运行的动力，气行则血行，气滞则血瘀。若肝失疏泄，气滞血瘀，则可见胸胁刺痛，甚至癥积、肿块，女子还可出现经行不畅、痛经和经闭等。

此外，肝的疏泄功能还有疏利三焦、通调水道的作用。故肝失疏泄，有时还可出现腹水、水肿等。

2) Storing and Regulating Blood

The liver has the function of storing blood and regulating its amount. When the human body is in the state of rest or sleep, it needs less blood, and most blood is stored in the liver. But when it is performing physical labour or working, the amount of blood needs to be increased. The liver will expel the blood it has stored, satisfying the need of the activities of the body. Modern physiology also believes that while a human is lying calmly, his whole liver system can store 55 percent of the total blood in his body. In the case of emergency a normal adult's liver can provide, at least, 1,000—2,000 milliliters of so as blood to keep enough blood for the heart to pump out. So it can be seen that the understanding of this function of the liver in both TCM and Western medicine is almost the same.

3) Having Relationship with Tendons, Nails and Eyes

The condition of the liver determines the condition of the tendons. The tendons depend on the nutrients from the blood of the liver to perform their functions., Malnutrition of the tendons due to the deficiency of blood from the liver may bring on numbness of the extremities, sluggishness of joint movement, spasm of the tendons and tremors of the hands and feet. Overabundance of pathogenic heat burns the *yin* of the liver, which results in spasms of the extremities, lockjaw, and opisthotonos. TCM calls this "liver-wind stirring inside". "Nails", in TCM, refer to the fingernails and toenails. TCM believes that nails and tendons have the same source of nutrients. So it is known that "The nail is the surplus of the tendon." The sufficiency of the blood of the liver gives ruddy, hard nails, but the deficiency of it results in withered, soft, thin or hollow and deformed nails.

"The liver has its specific body opening in the eyes." The eye's visual sense is mainly dependent on the nutrients from the blood of the liver to function well. The Liver Channel

2）主藏血

肝有贮藏血液和调节血量的功能。当人体在休息和睡眠时，机体的需血量减少，大量血液贮藏于肝；当劳动或工作时，机体的需血量增加，肝就排出其所储藏的血液，以供应机体活动的需要。现代生理学亦认为，人静卧时，整个肝脏系统可以贮藏全身血容量的55%；正常人一旦有紧急情况，肝脏至少能提供1,000～2,000毫升血液，以维持足够的心排出量。由此可见，中西医对肝这一功能的认识还是十分接近的。

3）肝与筋、爪、目的关系

肝主筋，筋的活动有赖于肝血的滋养。若肝血不足，筋失濡养，可出现肢体麻木、屈伸不利、筋脉挛急、手足震颤等症状，若热邪炽盛，燔灼肝的阴血，可出现四肢抽搐、牙关紧闭、角弓反张等，中医称之为“肝风内动”。中医所说的“爪”包括指甲和趾甲，中医认为爪甲的营养来源与筋相同，称为“爪为筋之余”。肝血充足，则指甲红润、坚韧；肝血不足，则爪甲枯槁、软薄，或凹陷变形。

“肝开窍于目”，目的视觉功能主要依赖肝之阴血的濡养；肝

goes upward to the eye system. Therefore, it is reflected in the eyes whether the liver's function is normal. For instance, the deficiency of the blood of the liver may lead to blurred vision and night blindness; the deficiency of the *yin* of the liver to dry eyes and hypopsia; the flaming up of excessive heat of the liver to red, sore, swollen eyes; bilirubinemia due to the dampness and heat in the liver and gallbladder to icteric sclera. In addition, there is also a saying that "Tears are the fluid of the liver."

Because the Liver Channel goes through hypochondria. lower abdomen and external genitals,diseases occurring in these organs should be treated by an overall analysis of signs and symptoms of the liver.

Note: From the physiology and pathology of the liver stated above, it can be seen the liver in TCM basically containts the functions of the liver that Western medicine deals with, part of the central nervous system, vegetative nervous system, blood and visual organ.

5. The Kidney

The kidney lies in the loins on either side of the spinal column. TCM classifies a kidney into the *yin* of the kidney (its material structures, including its essence of life) and the *yang* of the kidney (its funcetions and heat). The kidney essence of the life is stored within them. The *qi* of the kidney is produced by the kidney's essence of life. The following are the main functions of the kidney:

1) Storing the Essence of Life

The essence of life stored in the kidney is divided into two types.

(1) Congenital Essence of Life

This kind of essence of life is also known as "the essence of life from the kidney itself". It is inherited from the parents, and is enriched and strengthened by acquired food essence.

的经脉又上联目系。因此，肝的功能正常与否常常在目上反映出来。例如：肝血不足可出现视物模糊、夜盲；肝阴亏损，则两目干涩、视力减退；肝火上炎，可目赤肿痛；肝胆湿热，胆汁外溢，可出现巩膜黄染。此外，尚有“泪为肝之液”的说法。

肝的经脉循行于胁肋、小腹和外生殖器等部位，故这些部位的病症多从肝论治。

按语：从上述肝的生理、病理来看，中医的“肝”基本上包括了西医的肝以及部分中枢神经、植物神经、血液系统和视觉器官的功能。

5. 肾

肾位于腰部，脊柱两侧。中医将肾本身分为肾阴，即肾的物质与结构，包括肾精；肾阳，即肾的功能与热力；肾精，即肾所藏的精；肾气，由肾精所化生的“气”。肾的主要功能如下：

1）主藏精

肾所藏的精有以下两种：

(1)先天之精

又称肾本脏之精。这种肾精禀受于父母，来源于先天，并依

The essence of life can be transformed into *qi*.The *qi* transformed from the essence of life from the kidney is known as the *qi* of the kidney, which is the material basis on which the human body grows, develops and reproduces. For example, milk teeth are replaced by permanent teeth and hair grows longer when children are 7 or 8 years old. This is because the *qi* of their kidney is getting richer and richer. At the time when they reach the age of puberty, the *qi* of the kidney is richest. This causes their bodies to produce a substance called "*tian gui* in TCM". This substance not only promotes the development of sperm in boys, but also the discharge of eggs and menstruation in girls. The sexual function is perfected gradually till, at last, the ability to reproduce is fully developed. In old age, the *qi* of the kiduey becomes weak, which causes sexual functions and reproductive abilities to become ever weaker and then disappear. This is why TCM often utilizes the method of reinforcing the kidney to treat disorders such as slow development, premature senility and low sperm count in men, and delayed menstrual cycle or amenorrhea and primary sterility in women.

(2) Acquired Essence of Life

Acquired essence of life is also known as "five viscera and six bowels' essence of life". It is derived from food essence. Food essence is transformed by the spleen and stomach into the acquired essence of life, which is then transported to the five viscera and six bowels, coming to be the essence of life of viscera and bowels. When the essence of life of viscera and bowels is sufficient, part of it is provided for the needs of the physiological activities of the body, whereas the rest is stored in the kidney in preparation for future needs. Whenever the essence of life of viscera and bowels is not sufficient, the kidney will draw and send the essence of life it has stored to the five viscera and six bowels. Therefore, the richness or otherwise of the essence of life stored in the kidney is related to the functions of every viscus and bowel. TCM believes "When diseases of

靠后天水谷之精的滋养而充实、壮大。精能化气，肾精所化之气称为“肾气”。它是人体生长发育与生殖的物质基础。例如：人在七、八岁时，由于肾气的逐渐充盛，所以有“齿更发长”的变化；发育到青春时期，肾气充盛，产生了一种叫做“天癸”的物质，于是男子就能产生精子，女子就开始排卵，出现月经，性机能逐渐成熟而有生殖能力；待到老年，肾气渐衰，性机能和生殖能力随之逐渐减退而消失。故中医对发育迟缓和早衰、男性精液稀少、女子月经迟迟不来或闭经，或原发性不孕，多采用补肾法。

(2)后天之精

又称五脏六腑之精，后天之精来源于水谷精微，由脾胃化生，转输五脏六腑，成为脏腑之精。脏腑之精充盛，除供应本身生理活动所需外，其剩余部分则贮藏于肾，以备不时之需。当五脏六腑需要时，肾再把所藏的这些精气重新供给五脏六腑。故肾精的盛衰，对各脏腑的功能都有影响，中医有“五脏之病，穷必及肾”

all the other viscera are too severe, they are certain to involve the kidney." So, in the clinical treatment of prolonged diseases and severe deficiency of the heart, the liver, the spleen and the lung, what shonld always be considered is the inclusion of treatment of the kidney.

2) Regulating Water Metabolism

Regulating water metabolism is the function of the kidney, which regulates water circulation and helps maintain fluid balance in the body. Water metabolism of the human body has two aspects. One is to disseminate body fluid which has been derived from food essence and has nutritive and nourishing functions to the tissues, viscera and bowels throughout the body. The other is to discharge from the body the turbid fluid (waste) produced by all the viscera and bowels after metadolism. All these rely mainly on the kidney's function of regulating water metabolism.

The kidney has the function of controlling the opening and closing the gate of water. Opening the gate makes the water excreted, while closing the gate helps retain the water needed by the organ. If the function of regulating water metabolism is normal, opening or closing the gate of water will be properly regulated, resulting in normal urination. If this function is abnormal it can lead to inappropriate opening or closing of the gate of water, causing a backdown in the metabolism of watr. When closing occurs more often than opening, oliguria and edema occur. But when the reverse occurs, polyuria and frequent urination are apparent.

3) Controlling and Promoting Inspiration

TCM believes that although it is the lung that performs the function of respiration, the kidney can aid in inhaling the air downwards. This is known as "The kidney has the function of controlling and promoting inspiration." When the

的说法，所以临床上凡心、肝、脾、肺等脏病久或虚甚，都要考虑到治肾。

2）主水液

是指肾具有主持全身水液代谢、维持体内水液平衡的作用。人体的水液代谢包括两个方面：一是将来自水谷精微,具有濡养、滋润脏腑组织作用的津液输布全身；二是将各脏腑组织代谢后的浊液排出体外。而这些代谢过程的实现，主要依赖肾的“气化”功能。

肾有司开阖的作用。开，则水液得以排出；阖，则机体需要的水液能以在体内潴留。如果肾的气化正常，则开阖有度，尿液排泄也就正常。如果肾主水的功能失调，开阖失度，就会引起水液代谢紊乱。如阖多开少，可见尿少、水肿；开多阖少,则尿多、尿频。

3）主纳气

中医认为，人的呼吸虽由肺所主，但肾能帮助肺吸气下降，称为“肾主纳气”。如肾虚不能纳气，可出现呼多吸少、吸气困难、

kidney fails to do so because of a deficiency, expiration will occur more frequently than inspiration, as well as dyspnea and severe panting on moving. This is known as "The kidney fails to perform the function of controlling and promoting inspiration".

4) Determining the Condition of the Bone and Marrow, Having Its Manifestations in the Hair of the Head

The kidney stores the essence of life, which can be transformed into bone marrow. The bone marrow stored in the bone cavity nourishes the bone. This is known as "the condition of the kidney determining the condition of the bone", and "the kidney promoting the formation of bone marrow". The bone cavity is full of bone marrow if the essence of life stored in the kidney is sufficient. The bone is solid and strong if it is fully nourished by bone marrow. Not enough bone marrow is formed if the essence of life of the kidney is insufficient. An insufficiency of bone marrow can not nourish the bone fully. A malnourished bone is soft and weak, or even maldeveloped and, in babies, late closure of the fontanel and soft, weak bones often result from a deficiency of the essence of life of the kidney.

The teeth are also nourished by the kidney's essence of life, which is known as "the teeth being the surplus of the bone". So TCM believes that disorders such as slowly-growing teeth of children, loose or early loss of teeth of adults are manifestations of a deficiency of the essence of life of the kidney. Replenishing the kidney's essence of life should be used in the treatment of the above conditions.

Although the nutrients for hair come from the blood, its life mechanism originates from the kidney. This is because the kidney stores the essence of life and the essence of life can turn into blood. The flourishing and sufficient essence of life and blood lead to strong, bright hair. This is called, "The function of the kidney reflects in the glossiness of hair." Most people who have sparse or withered hair and / or loss of hair due

动则喘甚等症，称为“肾不纳气”。

4）主骨生髓，其华在发

肾藏精，精能生髓，髓藏于骨腔中以营养骨骼，称为“肾主骨”、“肾生骨髓”。肾精充足，则骨髓充盈。骨骼得到骨髓的充分滋养，才坚固有力。如果肾精虚少，骨髓的化源不足，不能营养骨骼，便会出现骨骼软弱无力，甚至发育不良，所以小儿囟门迟闭、骨软无力，常因肾精不足所致。

牙齿与骨一样，也是由肾精所充养，称为“齿为骨之余”。故凡小儿牙齿生长迟缓、成人牙齿松动或早期脱落，中医认为都是肾精不足的表现，治疗采用补益肾精法。

发的营养虽源于血，但其生机却根源于肾。因为肾藏精，精能化血，精血旺盛，则毛发壮而润泽，即所谓“其华在发”。凡久

to prolonged diseases, and those who are bald or have grey hair due to premature senility, are those who have been suffering from a lack of the kidney's essence of life and a deficiency of blood.

5) Having Its Specific Openings in the Ears and the Two "*Yin*" — Urinogenital Orifice and the Anus

The sense of hearing of the ears is detrermined by nourishment from the kidney's essence of life. Sufficient essence of life gives a keen sense of hearing. Otherwise, tinnitus and hypoacusis result.

Tne two *yin* means the front and back private parts. The private part includes the urethra and genitalia. Although urine is stored and eliminated by the urinary bladder, this process can not be fulfilled without the kidney's function of regulating water metabolism. This is why these disorders such as frequent urination, enuresis or oliguria and urodialysis are often related to the abnormal function of the kidney. As to the relationship between the kidney and the reproductive function, nothing will be added to what has been stated above.

The back private part refers to the anus. The large intestine controls the removal of feces. However, TCM believes that this also has something to do with the kidney. For example, a deficiency of the *yin* of the kidney may cause the intestinal juice to dry up, leading to constipation. A deficiency and weakness of the *yang* of the kidney presents a cold spleen and an accumulation of water and dampness. This may be a cause for loose stools. The *qi* of the kidney being not consolidated may result in loose stools over a long period or spontaneous defecation while eating.

Supplement: Vital Gate

The term "vital gate" appeared for the first time in the book ***Canon of Medicine***. But then it referred to the eyes and the point Jingming. For instance, the book "*Ling Shu•Gen*

病而见头发稀疏、枯槁、脱落，或未老先衰、早脱、早白者，多属肾精不足和血虚。

5）肾开窍于耳及二阴

耳的听觉功能依赖于肾精的充养。肾精充足，则听觉灵敏；肾精不足，则出现耳鸣、听力减退等。

二阴是前阴与后阴的总称。前阴包括尿道和生殖器。尿液的贮存和排泄虽是膀胱的功能，但须经肾的气化作用才能完成。因此，凡尿频、遗尿或尿少、闭尿多与肾的功能失常有关。至于肾与生殖机能的关系，已如前述，不再重赘。

后阴是指肛门。粪便的排泄虽由大肠所主，但中医认为亦与肾有关。如肾阴不足可致肠液枯涸而便秘；肾阳虚衰，脾失温煦，水湿不运，可致大便泄泻；肾气不固，可致久泄，滑脱。

附：命门

“命门”一词始见于《内经》，但它所说的命门是指的眼睛和睛明穴。如《灵枢·根结篇》说：“太阳根于至阴，结于命门。命门者，

Jie Pian", i.e., Points Where Channels Originate and End, a chapter of ***Miracvlous Pivot***, says, "The *Taiyang* Channel originates from the Point Zhiyin and ends at the vital gate. What the vital gate means is nothing but the eyes." It is the book ***Classic on Medical Problems*** that speaks, for the first time, of the vital gates as an internal organ. For instance, the chapter "Problem 36" (The 36th Medical Problem) says, "It is known to all that there are two kidneys in the human body. But in fact both of them are not kidneys. The left one is the kidney, while the right one is the vital gate." The medical men of later generations have different opinions on the identity and functions of the vital gate. For instance, Zhang Jiebin in the Ming dynasty said, "The vital gate is both the root of the inborn *qi* and the house of water and fire. The *yin* of the five viscera has to depend on it for nutrients. The *yang* of the five viscera has to depend on it for developing". That is, he thought the functions of the vital gate are equal to those of both the *yin* and *yang* of the kidney. However, Zhao Xianke in the Ming dynasty proposed that the vital gate lies in the portion between the two kidneys and the fire of the vital gate is nothing but the *yang* of the human body. From TCM's clinical observations it is found that diseases due to the decline of the fire from the vital gate are basically similar to those due to a deficiency of the *yang* of the kidney, and most drugs used to reinforce the fire of the vital gate have the function of replenishing the *yang* of the kidney. This points to the fire of the vital gate being basically the same as the *yang* of the kidney. The term "vital gate" is used to emphasize the importance of the *yang* of the kidney.

Note: From the kidney's physiology and pathology stated above we can see that the kidney in TCM basically includes the functions of the urinary system, reproductive system, and part of the endocrine system and nervous system.

In the light of research on the kidney by a special group

目也。”将命门作为内脏提出，则始于《难经》，如《三十六难》说：“肾两者，非皆肾也，其左者为肾，右者为命门。”后世医家对命门的部位及其功能有不同的认识。如明代张介宾说：“命门为元气之根，为水火之宅，五脏之阴气非此不能滋，五脏之阳气非此不能发。”即认为命门的功能包括肾阴、肾阳两个方面的作用。但明代赵献可则提出命门的部位在“两肾之间”，认为命门火即人体阳气。从中医临床角度看，命门火衰所出现的病症与肾阳不足的病症多属一致，治疗时所用的补命门火的药物，又多具有补肾阳的作用。因此，可以认为，命门火与肾阳基本相同，之所以称为“命门”，无非是强调肾阳的重要性而已。

按语：从上述肾的生理、病理看来，中医的肾基本上包括了现代医学的泌尿、生殖系统以及部分内分泌、神经系统的功能。

据上海第一医学院脏象专题研究组有关肾的研究，发现六种

at The First Medical College in Shanghai who studied this organ, it has been found that any of the following six different diseases: anovulatory and functional uterine bleeding, bronchial asthma, toxemia of pregnancy, coronary atherosclerotic heart disease, lupus erythematosus and neurasthenia, is present with low 17-hydroxycorticosteriod if the *yang* of the kiney is diagnosed to be deficient. After a test in which adrenocorticotropic hormone was given by intravenous injection for two days, delayed reactions occured among half of the patients whose *yang* of the kidney was deficient. This test reveals a subnormal excitability of the system of the pituitary body — adrenal cortex in the patient whose *yang* of the kidney is deficient. Based on this assumption, another clinical test was made. The method of reinforcing the essence of the kidney was tried in treating the patients with asthma who depended on taking cortical hormone over a long period of time and whose reserving function of the pituitary body was subnormal without the symptoms of a deficiency of the kidney. A curative effect became apparent which seemed to verify, at an elementary level, the assumption of the researchers.

Section 2

Six Bowels (*Fu*-organ)

1. The Gallbladder

The gallbladder is attached to the liver. It is a hollow capsule-shaped organ. Its main functions are as follows:

1) Storing and Excreting Bile

Bile is made and secreted by the liver. Then it goes into the gallbladder and is stored and concentrated there. Finally it is pumped into the small intestine by the liver's function of smoothing and regulating the flow of the *qi* in promoting the di-

不同的疾病(无非卵性功能性子宫出血、支气管哮喘、妊娠中毒症、冠状动脉粥样硬化性心脏病、红斑性狼疮、神经衰弱)凡辨证为肾阳虚者，均有尿17羟皮质类固醇值低下的现象，在采用促肾上腺皮质激素静脉滴注试验2日后，发现肾阳虚病人半数有延迟反应，提示肾阳虚病人有垂体—肾上腺皮质系统兴奋性低下。一以此假定再试用于临床，对虽无明显肾虚症状的肾上腺皮质储备功能低下及长期用激素不易撤去的哮喘患者采用补肾治疗，获得显著疗效，说明这一假定得到了实践的初步验证。

第二节　六　腑

1. 胆

胆附于肝，是一中空囊状器官。其主要功能如下：

1) 贮藏、排泄胆汁

胆汁由肝脏制造、分泌，然后进入胆贮存、浓缩，并通过肝的疏泄作用注入小肠，以促进食物的消化、吸收。若肝胆功能失

gestion and absorption of food. If the functions of the liver and gallbladder are abnormal, and the secretion and excretion of bile is obstructed, the digestion and absorption of food will be disturbed, which results in loss of appetite, distension of the epigastrium and diarrhea. The accumulation of pathogenic damp-heat in the liver and gallbladder impairs the liver's function of smoothing and regulating the flow of *qi* and causes bile to overflow to muscle and skin, which will lead to jaundice which is manifested as icteric sclera, yellowish skin, yellow urine and so on. The boring of round worms into the biliary tract results in paroxysmal angina in the right upper quadrant of the abdomen or in the area under the ensiform process slightly inclining to the right. This is what is called in TCM, "colic caused by ascaris marked by abdominal paroxysmal colic pains with cold limbs".

2) Having Something to Do with One's Courage in Making Decisions

The Functions of the Viscera and Bowels, a chapter of ***Plain Questions***, says, "The gallbladder seems to be an upright officer who is in charge of making a decision." This gives its idea that the gallbladder is concerned with one's courage in making decisions, i.e., bravery and timidity are related to the gallbladder. From then on, TCM began to diagnose and treat pathological changes in mind, such as being easily frightened and scared, insomnia, dream-disturbed sleep and so on, by an overall analysis of signs and symptoms concerned with the gallbladder.

Although the gallbladder is among the six bowels, it simply stores bile, and does not receive any water, food or waste. This makes it different from the other five bowels. Hence it also comes under "extraordinary organs".

Note: From the physiology and pathology of the gallbladder stated above, it can be seen that TCM observes the gallbladder

常，胆汁的分泌、排泄障碍，可影响食物的消化、吸收，从而出现厌食、腹胀和腹泄等。若湿热蕴结肝胆，以致肝失疏泄，胆汁外溢肌肤，则发为黄疸，表现为目黄、身黄、小便黄等。蛔虫钻入胆道，可引起右上腹或剑突下略偏右阵发性绞痛，中医称之为“蛔厥”。

2）主决断

《素问·灵兰秘典论》云：“胆者，中正之官，决断山焉。”即认为人的勇、怯与胆有关。故中医对胆怯易惊、善恐、失眠、多梦等神志病变，常从胆论治。

胆虽为六腑之一，但其藏胆汁，并不接受水谷或糟粕，与其他五腑不同，故又被归属于“奇恒之腑”。

按语：从上述胆的生理、病理看，中医对胆的认识与西医基

basically in the same way as Western medicine except that it takes some of the functions of the partial nervons system for the gallbladder's.

2. The Stomach

The stomach lies under the diaphragm in the upper part of the abdominal cavity. Its upper opening connects with the esophagus. Its lower opening is the pylorus which connects with the small intestine. TCM names the upper part of the stomach "*shang wan*", which includes the cardia; the lower parts is named "*xia wan*", which includes the pylorus. The area between "*shang wan*" and "*xie wan*" is known as "*zhong wan*". All three parts are collectively known as "*wei wan*".

The stomach's main physiological function is to receive, digest and transform water and food. Diet enters the mouth, passes through the esophagus, reaches the stomach and remains there. This is why the stomach is called "the reservoir of water and food". The water and food held in the stomach is reduced to chyme by the fermenting and grinding action of the stomach. Then the chyme is forced downward into the small intestine. A disturbance of this function of the stomach will cause poor appetite, a capacity for only small amount of food, indigestion and distension and pain in the epigastric region. Of course, only in cooperation with the spleen's function of transportation and transformation can the stomach's function of receiving, digesting and transforming water and food be performed successfully. How right Cheng Wuji (1062—1155 A.D.) was when he said, "It seems as if the spleen is the earth, which helps the *qi* of the stomach to grind and digest water and food. When the *qi* of the spleen failed to transport and transform, the water and food in the stomach would remain unchanged."

TCM attaches great importance to the *qi* of the stomach, and believes "A human body's essence is the *qi* of the stomach." A sufficiency of *qi* of the stomach causes all five viscera to be full

本相同，但将部分神经系统的某些功能亦归属于胆。

2. 胃

胃位于膈下，腹腔上部。其上口名贲门，与食道相接；下口名幽门，与小肠相通。中医将胃的上部名“上脘”，包括贲门；下部名“下脘”，包括幽门；上，下脘之间名“中脘”。三部统称为“胃脘”。

胃的主要生理功能是受纳、腐熟水谷。饮食入口，经过食道，容纳于胃，故称胃为“水谷之海”。容纳于胃的水谷，通过胃的腐熟、消磨，形成食糜，并下移于小肠。如果胃的这一功能障碍，可出现食欲不振、食量减少、消化不良、胃脘胀痛等。当然，胃受纳、腐熟水谷的功能，必须与脾的运化功能相配合，才能顺利完成。如成无己说：“脾，坤土也。坤助胃气，消磨水谷。脾气不转，则胃中水谷不得消磨。”

中医十分重视“胃气”，认为“人以胃气为本”，胃气强则五脏

of vigour, while a deficiency leads to their weakness. While the *qi* of the stomach exists, life continues; without it, life comes to an end. By the *qi* of the stomach we mean, on the one hand, the physiological functions of the stomach and, on the other hand, how the spleen and stomach work on the pulse, securing a pulse condition of being gentle but strong, not too fast and not too slow.

It is normal for the *qi* of the stomach to descend. After being digested and transformed by the stomach, the food content follows the *qi* of the stomach down into the small intestine so as to undergo further digestion and absorption. If the *qi* of the stomach ascends instead of descending, belching, hicups, nausea or vomiting will occur.

The stomach belongs to *yang* and has the characteristic of liking to be moistened but hating to be dried. Too excessive an amount of *yang* often brings on dryness and fire, whose manifestations are feeling dry in the mouth and thirst, dry and yellow coated tongue or gingival swelling and pain.

Note: From the stomach's physiology and pathology stated above, it can be seen that TCM has almost the same understanding of the stomach as Western medicine.

3. The Small Intestine

The small intestine is between the stomach and the large intestine. The section by which it is connected with the stomach is the pylorus. The section by which it is connected with the large intestine is "*lan men*" (the ileocecal region). The following are the main functions of the small intestine.

1) Receiving, Transforming and Absorbing the Food Content

The Functions of The Viscera and Bowels, a chapter of ***Plain Questions*** says, "The small intestine is like an officer who takes charge of receiving and then transforming things." In

盛，胃气弱则五脏俱衰；有胃气则生，无胃气则死。所谓胃气，一是指胃的生理功能，二是脾胃功能在脉象上的反映，即和缓有力、不快不慢之脉。

胃气宜降。饮食物经胃腐熟后，随其气下降而入小肠，以便使食物得到进一步地消化、吸收。如果胃气不降而反上逆，可出现嗳气、呃逆、恶心、呕吐等。

胃属阳，有"喜润恶燥"的特性，常因阳气过盛而形成燥火，出现口干喜饮、舌苔干黄或齿龈肿痛等。

按语，从上述胃的生理、病理看，中医对胃的认识与西医基本一致。

3. 小　肠

小肠上触胃，下触大肠。其与胃相接处名幽门，与大肠相接处名阑门。

小肠的主要生理功能如下：

2）主受盛化物

《素问·灵兰秘典论》说："小肠者，受盛之官，化物出焉。"

other words, the small intestine receives the food content which has been elementarily digested by the stomach, and then digests and absorbs it. Its dysfunction in doing this will lead to disorders in digestion and absorption manifested as abdominal distension, diarrhea, loose stools and others.

2) Separating Clarity from Turbidity

Separating clarity from turbidity means that having digested the food content fully, the small intestine sends the useful part (clarity) to the spleen, which in turn, transports and distributes it to all parts of the body. It also sends waste (turbidity) down into the large intestine through *lan men* (the ileocecal region); and sends unwanted water into the urinary bladder to be excreted from the body. When this function of the small intestine is normal, water and waste are excreted from the body separately, with smooth urination and normal elimination of feces. When the small intestine fails to separate the clarity from the turbidity, they will be mixed together, and water will be contained in the wastes, thus leading to dysuria and loose stools. TCM doctors often adopt the method of "treating diarrhea with diurectics."

Note: From the physiology and pathology of the small intestine stated above, it can be seen that TCM has almost the same knowledge of the small intestine as Western medicine.

4. The Large Intestine

The upper part of the large intestine is connected to the small intestine, and the lower part to the anus. Its main physiological function is to pass and eliminate waste, i.e., to receive the contents of the small intestine and absorb excessive water from it so that it forms feces which is discharged from the body through the anus. This is why The Functions of the Viscera and Bowels, a chapter of ***Plain Questions*** says, "It seems as if the large intestine served as the officer who was in charge of passing

是指小肠接受由胃初步消化的饮食物，并对其作进一步的消化、吸收。如这一功能异常，可导致消化、吸收障碍，表现为腹胀、腹泻、便溏等。

2）主泌别清浊

所谓泌别清浊，是说小肠将饮食物经过充分消化后，其精微物质由脾转送全身；其渣滓（浊）则通过“阑门”下注大肠；其无用之水液渗入膀胱，排出体外。小肠这一功能正常，则水液、糟粕各走其道，小便通利，大便正常；若小肠泌别失职，则清浊不分，水液归于糟粕，出现小便不利、大便溏泄等。中医治疗常用利小便即所以实大便的方法。

按语：从上述小肠的生理、病理看，中医对小肠的认识，与西医相似。

4．大 肠

大肠上接小肠，下接肛门，其主要生理功能是传导糟粕。即大肠接受由小肠下注的内容物，吸收多余的水分，使之形成大便，并经肛门排出体外。故《素问·灵兰秘典论》说：“大肠者，传导之官，变化出焉。”如传导失常，可出现大便质、量以及次数

and removing things." Its dysfunction may result in abnormal changes in ubstance and amount of feces and also times of difecation. For instance, a cold-deficiency of the large intestine causes it to be unable to absorb water so that water and wastes are removed together. This is manifested as diarrhea, borborygmus and abdominal pain. The sthenic heat of the large intestine consumes water,dries up the intestinal juice, resulting in constipation. The accumulation of damp-heat in the large intestine blocks the passage of *qi*, which leads to abdominal pain, tenesmus and stools with pus and blood.

Note: From the physiology and pathology of the large intestine stated above, it can be seen that TCM has almost the same knowledge of the large intestine as Western medicine.

5. The Urinary Bladder

The urinary bladder lies in the hypogastrium, under the kidney and in front of the large intestine, Its upper part is connected to the kidney by the ureters. Its lower part is connected to the urethra which opens externally by means of the urinary orifice.

The urinary bladder's main function is to store and excrete urine. In the course of water metabolism of the human body, the water is dissipated to all parts of the body by the action of the lung, the spleen and the kidney thereby fulfilling its function of moistening the body. After being utilized by the body it accumulates in the kidney. There, it is decomposed into two parts, the clarity and the turbidity by means of the kidney's function of separating the clear fluid from the turbid. Clear fluid is delivered back to the whole body. Turbid fluid is changed into urine and transported down into the urinary bladder. There, when urine amounts to a certain quantity, the urinary bladder excretes it from the body voluntarily and on time. So the Functions of Viscera and Bowels, a chapter of the medical classic ***Plain Questions*** says, "The urinary bladder

的异常变化。如大肠虚寒，无力吸收水分，水谷杂下，可出现泄泻、肠鸣、腹痛等：大肠实热，消烁水分，肠液干枯，可出现大便秘结不通；湿热蕴结大肠，大肠气滞，可出现腹痛、里急后重、便脓血等。

按语：从上述大肠的生理、病理看，中医对大肠的认识与西医十分接近。

5. 膀胱

膀胱位于下腹部，居肾之下，大肠之前。其上有输尿管与肾相通，其下有尿道，开口于前阴，称为尿窍。

膀胱的主要生理功能是贮藏、排泄尿液。在人体水液代谢过程中，水液通过肺、脾、肾等脏的作用，布散全身，发挥润泽机体的作用。其被人体利用之后，下归于肾，经过肾的气化作用，升清降浊，其清者回流体内，浊者变成尿液，下输膀胱，当其达到一定容量时，通过膀胱的气化功能及时而自主地将尿液排出体

serves as the officer of an administrative division who takes charge of storing and excreting water (urine)." A dysfunction of the urinary bladder in storing and excreting urine may result in dysuria or retention of urine. That the urinary bladder fails to store urine may lead to frequent micturition and incontinence of urine. The dampness and heat accumulated in the urinary bladder often causes frequent micturition, urgent urination and pain in micturition.

TCM believes that the fulfillment of the urinary bladder's function of storing and excreting urine depends on the aid of the kidney's function of dividing the clear fluid from the turbid. This is why a patient who has enuresis and incontinence of urine is often treated by means of replenishing the kidney.

Note: From the physiology and pathology of the urinary bladder stated above, it can be seen that TCM has basically the same knowledge of the urinary bladder as Western medicine.

6. The Triple Warmer (*Sanjiao*)

The term, triple warmer, is peculiar to TCM. It is a collective name of the upper, middle and lower warmer and is one of the six bowels. In the field of TCM, no unanimous conclusion has been drawn about the form and crux of the triple warmer. It is generally recognized that "triple warmer" is a large bowel containing all the internal organs. For instance, Zhang Jiebin, a medical man in the Ming dynasty, said "Triple warmer is,in fact, a bowel. It is outside all the viscera and bowels but within the body, contain all the other organs and is the largest bowel within the body cavity." In the theory of TCM the term "triple warmer" is also used to locate the body parts. The upper warmer (*jiao*) is that the portion of the body cavity above the diaphragm which houses the heart and the lung. The middle warmer (*jiao*) is the portion between the diaphragm and umbilicus which houses the spleen and the stomach. The lower warmer (*jiao*) is the portion below the umbilicus which

外。故《素问·兰秘典论》说："膀胱者，州都之官，津液藏焉，气化则能出矣。"如膀胱气化不行，可见小便不利或癃闭；膀胱失其约束，则见尿频、小便失禁；膀胱湿热，常见尿频、尿急、尿痛等。

中医认为，膀胱的贮尿、排尿功能，有赖肾脏气化功能的帮助才能完成。故对遗尿、小便失禁的病人，常以补肾为法。

按语：从上述膀胱的生理、病理看，中医对膀胱的认识与西医大致相同。

6. 三 焦

三焦，是中医脏腑学说中一个特有的名词。三焦是上焦、中焦、下焦的合称，为六腑之一。关于三焦的形态与实质，中医界众说纷纭，至今尚无定论。一般认为，三焦是包罗人体所有内脏的一个大腑，如明·张介宾说："三焦者，确有一腑，盖脏腑之外，躯壳之内，包罗诸脏，一腔之大腑也。"在中医理论中，三焦也是划分躯体部位的一个概念。即膈以上的部位为上焦，包括心、肺；

houses the liver, the kidney, the urinary bladder, the intestines and the uterus. According to the liver's location, it can be clearly seen that the liver is an organ within the middle warmer. But it is said that the liver is an organ within the lower warmer. Why? Because TCM believes the liver and the kidney have the same source and a close relationship, and this puts the liver into the lower warmer.

Generally speaking, the physiological functions of triple warmer control the activities of the *qi* of the human body. The upper warmer controls respiration, and activates the flow of vital energy, blood and body fluid (referring to in fact, the functions of the heart and lung), i.e., it disperses pectoral *qi* accumulated in the chest to all parts of the body just as fog and dew moisten the earth. This is why TCM says that "The upper warmer is like a sprinkler for distributing nutrients and *qi*." The middle warmer functions in transportation and transformation(referring to in fact, the functions of the spleen and stomach), i.e. it ferments water and food and transports and transforms food essence in order to produce vital energy and blood. Therefore, it is likened to a fermentation tun, where food is digested. The lower warmer separates clear fluid from turbid fluid and discharges urine and stool, (referring to, in fact, the functions of the kidney ,the small intestine, the large intestine and the urinary bladder). These two physiological functions mentioned above are characterised by excreting wastes downwards and outwards. It is said that the lower warmer works like gutters, to filter and drain off waste and superfluous water. In fact, all these physiological functions of the triple warmer are the sum total of the activities of all the viscera and bowels in the body. Pathologically, diseases due to an abnormality of upper, or middle, or lower warmer are manifestations of dysfunctions of the viscera or bowels within it.

TCM also believes that the triple warmer is the passage through which water, food and fluid are transported. For

膈以下、脐以上的部位为中焦，包括脾、胃；脐以下为下焦，包括肝、肾、大小肠、膀胱、女子胞等。其中肝脏，按其部位来说，应划归中焦。但中医认为，肝肾同源，关系密切，故将肝肾同划归下焦。

三焦的生理功能，总的来说，是总司人体气化。分开来说，上焦主呼吸、主宣发（实指心、肺的功能），即把积于胸中的“气”宣布、布达全身，若雾露之溉，故称“上焦如雾”；中焦主运（实指脾、胃的功能），即腐熟水谷，运化精微，以化气血，故喻之为“中焦如沤”；下焦主分别清浊、排泄尿液与大便（实指肾、小肠、大肠、膀胱的功能），以上生理功能均具有向下、向外排泄的特点，故称“下焦如渎”。三焦的这些生理功能，实际上是体内各脏腑功能的总合。在病理上，上、中、下三焦异常所出现的病证，实际上也是各部位脏腑功能的异常表现。

中医还认为，三焦是水谷、水液运行的道路。如《难经》说：

instance, the book ***Classic on Medical Problems*** says, "The triple warmer is the passage for water and food to follow." The book ***Canon of Medicine*** says, "The triple warmer may be compared to water communications. It is the foundation and controller of the entire circulation of body fluid." All these functions result from the comprehensive action of the lung, the spleen, the kidney and so on. This is why difficult urination and edema due to an abnormality in the triple warmer and the blocking of water passages are treated by recuperating the lung, the spleen and the kidney.

In addition, in the course of diagnosing and treating febrile diseases by differentiation of syndromes, the theory of triple warmer is used to guide the classfication of the three different portions of the body—the upper, middle and lower — through which the pathogenic noxious factors make their invasion. In addition, it serves to determine the three different phases of the development of epidemic febrile diseases — the primary, intermediate and last. It is based on this theory that "a dialectical method" of analysing and differentiating diseases according to the pathological changes of triple warmer is formed.

Section 3
Extraordinary Organs

TCM recognizes the brain, the medulla, the bones, the blood vessels, the gallbladder and the uterus collectively as the "extraordinary organs". Included is the gallbladder which is also one of the six bowels and has been dealt with previously. The blood vessels, the medulla and the bones were also introduced when speaking of the heart and the kidney of the five viscera. Here only TCM's understanding of the brain and the uterus will be discussed.

"三焦者，水谷之道路"；《内经》云："三焦者，决渎之官，水道出焉。"这些功能实际上是肺、脾、肾等脏腑功能的综合作用。故对三焦异常，水道不通，出现小便不利或水肿，仍以调治肺、脾、肾为主。

此外，在温病的辨施治证中，三焦又是划分病邪侵入人体上中下三个不同部位和温病发展过程中初、中、末三个不同阶段的一种分类方法，即"三焦辨证法"。

第三节 奇恒之腑

中医将脑、髓、骨、脉、胆、女子胞统称为奇恒之腑。其中，胆亦为六腑之一，前面已作论述；脉、髓、骨也已在五脏之心、肾中作了介绍，故概不重赘。这里仅就中医对脑、女子胞的认识论述如下：

1. The Brain

Marrow combines to form the brain, which is contained in the cranial cavity. So The Seas in the Human Body, a chapter of the medical classic ***Miraculous Pivot***, says, "The brain is a sea of marrow." The main functions of the brain are as follows:

1) Controlling Mental and Thinking Activities

TCM has long understood the relationship between the brain and mental and reasoning activities. For example, The Essence of Sphygmology, a chapter of the ***Plain Ouestions*** says, "The head is the source of mental activities." In the Qing dynasty, Wang Ang, a medical man, wrote a book entitled Essential of Materia Medica, in which there is a clear-cut sentence "A person's memory is wholly stored in the brain." Later, Wang Qingren, a medical man also in the Qing dynasty, stated clearly, "The spirit and memory are not stored in the heart but in the brain." This shows that the brain operates mental activities.

2) Guiding Sensuous and Language Activities

As early as the time when the "***Canon of Medicine***" was written, TCM associated the audio and visual senses with the brain. In the Qing dynasty, Wang Qingren pointed out, "The two ears are linked to the brain, and a sound that the ears receive are transmitted into it. The eyes are connected by lineal things to the brain, which receive an image the eyes catch. The nose is linked to the brain, to which goes the sweet or foul odour the nose smells. A one-year old baby can say one word or two, because its brain has been growing gradually." In his book, he attributed the functions of seeing, hearing, smelling and speaking to the brain. Of all the books on TCM, his deals most comprehensively with the functions of the brain.

1. 脑

脑位于颅腔内，由髓汇集而成，故《灵枢·海伦》说："脑为髓之海。"脑的主要功能如下：

1）主精神、思维

中医对脑与精神、思维活动的关系早有认识。如《素问·脉要精微论》说："头者，精明之府。"至清代汪昂之《本草备要》更有"人之记性，皆在脑中"的记载。其后，清·王清任则明确提出："灵机、记性不在心，在脑。"以上均说明脑有主持精神、思维活动的功能。

2）主感觉、语言

早在《内经》时代，中医就已把视觉、听觉与脑联系在一起了。至清代王清任更明确指出："两耳通脑，所听之音归脑；两目系如线长于脑，所见之物归脑；鼻通于脑，所闻香臭归于脑；小儿周岁脑渐生，舌能言一、二字。"他把视、听、嗅、言等感觉和语言统属于脑，是中医书籍中言脑功能最全者。

Although TCM has had certain knowledge of the brain's physiology and pathology, it still believes that most mental, conscious and reasoning activities result separately from the five viscera and the gallbladder. The theory of viscera and bowels says that the heart houses the mind and ensures the existence of pleasure. The lung stores the inferior spirit and causes sorrow when it has problems. The spleen houses intentions and takes part in directing reasoning. The liver stores the soul and its disorder may cause anger. The kidney stores the memory and its disorder may cause fright. The gallbladder is associated with one's courage in making decisions. Among these, the heart, the liver and the kidney play the major part in controlling mental activities. Therefore, in TCM, either syndromes established by an overall differentiation of the signs and symptoms of diseases such as "the heart confused by phlegm", the stagnance of *qi* (vital energy) of the liver" and "the imbalance of the normal physiological coordination between the heart and the kidney" or their corresponding therapies, such as "resolving phlegm so as to open the aperture of the heart", "removing stagnance of vital energy of the liver in order to restore the normal function of a depressed liver" and "restoring balanced vital function of the heart and the vital essence of the kidney", are, in fact, included in Western medicine.

Note: From the foregoing physiology and pathology of the brain, it can be seen that although TCM is similar to Western medicine in understanding the brain in some aspects, there are different ways and depths in doing so.

2. The Uterus

The uterus lies in the lower abdomen of the female behind the urinary bladder and in front of the rectum. Its lower opening is connected to the vagina. Its shape is like an inverted pear. It is a reproductive organ of the female. Its main functions are as follows:

尽管中医对脑的生理、病理有了一定认识，但在中医脏腑学说中，却多把精神、意识、思维活动分别归属于五脏及胆。如提出心藏神，主喜；肺藏魄，主悲；脾藏意，主思；肺藏魂，主怒；肾藏志，主恐；胆主决断等。其中，尤以心、肝、肾为主。因而中医在辨证上之"痰迷心窍"、"肝气郁结"、"心肾不交"等证型，以及与此相应的"化痰开窍"、"疏肝解郁"、"交通心肾"等治法，实际上包括了西医脑的病症与治法。

按语：从上述脑的生理、病理看，中医对脑的认识虽某些地方与西医相近，但在认识方法及深度上，却有着质的区别。

2. 女子胞

女子胞位于小腹内，在膀胱之后，直肠之前，下口与阴道相通，呈倒置的梨形。它是女性的生殖器官，其主要功能如下：

1) Producing Menses

The uterus is the organ by which a woman forms menstruation. Generally speaking, a girl's *qi* of the kidney is increasing and her womb is fully developed when she reaches the age of 14 or so. Under the action of a substance named "*tian gui*", her *Ren* Channel flourishes to become more unobstructed, her *Chong* Channel flourishes more, her sea of blood becomes fuller, and she begins to have regular menses. When she becomes a woman of 49 years old, her *qi* of the kidney becomes weaker. The "*tian gui*" in her body is used up. Both her *Ren* and *Chong* Channels close and become obstructed and she begins to have menstrual disorders until menopause occurs.

2) Being Pregnant

Once a woman's uterus is fully developed and her menses are regular an egg from her ovary can be fertilized with sperm and pregnancy can result.

TCM believes the physiological functions of the woman's uterus are mainly related to the heart, the liver, the spleen, the kidney as well as the *Ren* Channel and the *Chong* Channel. This is because the functions of producing menses and becoming pregnant are not irrelative to the blood and the productive essence and, what is more, the heart controls blood circulation, the liver installs and regulates the blood, the spleen keeps the blood flowing within the vessels, the kidney stores the reproductive essence, and two channels mentioned above supply the uterus with the blood. Therefore, pathologically, abnormal functions of the above organs and channels caused by various pathogenic factors will affect the functions of the uterus, resulting in menstrual disorder and sterility. In the treatment of these disorders, TCM often begins with adjusting and replenishing the above organs.

Note: From the foregoing physiology and pathology of

1）主持月经

女子胞是女子形成月经的器官。女子一般到了14岁左右，肾气逐渐充盛，子宫发育成熟，在天癸的作用下，任脉通，冲脉盛，血海满盈，月经开始按时来潮；到了49岁左右，肾气渐衰，天癸枯竭，冲任二脉闭塞，逐渐出现月经紊乱，乃至绝经。

2）孕育胎儿

女子胞一旦发育成熟，月经按时来潮，就已具备了孕育胎儿的能力。如阴阳相合，就能有子。

中医认为，女子胞的生理功能主要与心、肝、脾、肾以及冲任二脉有关。这是因为其主持月经、孕育胎儿的功能无不与血、精有关，而心主血，肝藏血，脾统血，肾藏精，任主胎胞，冲为血海。在病理上，当各种因素导致上述脏器、经脉功能异常，即影响女子胞的功能，引起月经失调与不孕。因而在治疗上，中医多从调补以上脏器、经脉入手。

按语：从上述女子胞的生理、病理看，中医的女子胞不仅是

the uterus, it can be seen that the uterus in TCM refers not only to the womb but also to the whole internal genital system.

Section 4

The Relationship between Internal Organs

1. The Relationship between Viscera

The relationship between viscera means the interrelationship between the five viscera. In ancient times TCM always applied the theory of generation and restriction of the five elements to explain the physiological relations between the five viscera, and the theory of subjugation and reverse restriction of the five elements to explain the physiological influence between the five viscera. But, in fact, the generation, restriction, subjugation and reverse restriction of the theory of the five elements are not enough to explain the complex relations between the five viscera. Here the interrelationship between the five viscera will be discussed with emphasis on their physiological relationship and pathological influence.

1) The Relationship between the Heart and the Lung

The heart and the lung are both in the upper warmer. The heart controls the circulation of blood. The lung controls *qi*. The heart and the lung depend on each other for their existence, so do the circulation of blood and the *qi*. Blood circulation relies on the driving force of the *qi*. Meanwhile the *qi* needs the circulation of blood to transport and distribute it. Pathologically, a deficiency of the *qi* (functional activites) of the lung and a lack of pectoral *qi* (food energy plus cosmic energy) will lead to a lack of force to propel blood forward and then, to the stagnation of blood, thus causing a stuffy feeling

指子宫，而且还包含着整个女性内生殖系统。

第四节　脏腑之间的关系

1．脏与脏的关系

脏与脏之间的关系，即五脏之间的关系。在古代，中医多是以五行的相生、相克理论来解释五脏之间的生理联系，用五行的相乘、相侮来说明五脏之间的病理影响。但事实上，五脏之间的复杂关系早已超过了五行生、克、乘、侮的范围。因此，这里着重从各脏间的生理联系及其病理影响来阐述它们之间的相互关系。

1）心与肺

心、肺同居上焦。心主血，肺主气。心与肺，血与气，是相互依存的。血的运行有赖于气的推动，而气的输布也需要血的运载。在病理上，肺气虚弱，宗气不足，则运血无力，循行瘀阻，

in the chest, shortness of breath, palpitation, cyanosis of the lips and a purplish tongue. A deficiency of the *qi* of the heart and the stagnation of blood may affect the lung's function of dispersing and descending, thus causing cough, asthmatic breathing, shortness of breath, and stuffy feeling in the chest.

2) The Relationship between the Heart and the Spleen

The heart controls the circulation of blood. The spleen has the functions of producing blood and keeping it flowing within the vessels. The relationship between the heart and the spleen is mainly shown in the production and circulation of blood. Physiologically, if the spleen functions well both in transporting and distributing nutrients and water, and in providing sufficient nutrients for growth and development, the blood of the heart will be plentiful. A plentiful supply of blood of the heart will, in turn, provide the spleen with sufficient nutrients from the blood, and the spleen will function well in transporting and distributing nutrients and water. The flowing of blood through the vessels depends, not only on the driving force of the *qi* (functional activities) of the heart, but also on the function of the *qi* of the spleen in keeping the blood flowing within the vessels. Pathologically an insufficiency of the blood of the heart may result from a dysfunction of the spleen in transporting and distributing nutrients and water, inadequate nutrients for growth and development or a dysfunction of the spleen in keeping the blood flowing within the vessels and the extravasation of blood from the vessels. The spleen's function of transporting, distributing and transforming nutrients and promoting water metabolism may be affected by mental anxiety and an insufficiency of blood and *qi* (functional activities) of the heart. An insufficiency of the blood of the heart and a dysfunction of the spleen in transportation and transformation can cause signs and symptoms such as palpitation, insomnia, anorexia, lassitude and pallor. This is known in TCM as "a

从而出现胸闷、气短、心悸、唇青舌紫等；如心气不足，血运不畅，亦可影响肺的宣降功能，出现咳嗽、喘息、气促、胸闷等。

2）心与脾

心主行血，脾主生血、统血，心与脾的关系主要表现在血的生成与运行两个方面。在生理上，脾气健运，化源充足，则心血充盈；心血旺盛，脾得濡养，则脾气健运。血液在脉中循行，既赖心气的推动，又赖脾气的统摄。在病理上，脾失健运，化源不足，或脾不统血，血液外溢，均可致心血不足；而思虑过度，耗伤心血、心气，又可影响脾的运化。这些都会出现心悸、失眠、食少、

deficiency of both the heart and the spleen". To treat it, spleen-invigorating-and-heart-nourishing pills, such as *Gui Pi* Pill, are often used.

3) The Relationship between the Heart and the Liver

The heart is believed to be in charge of mental activities. The liver has the function of smoothing and regulating the fiow of *qi* and blood. They are both related to mental activities and mood. Pathologically, they affect each other as well. For example, a patient with harassment of deficient fire inside due to the deficiency of heart-*yin* may present the signs and symptoms of heart trouble such as upset, insomnia and dreaminess as well as those of liver trouble such as fidgetiness, easy anger and others. The patient with sthenic liver-*yang* may have the signs and symptoms of liver trouble, e.g., dizziness, a sensation of distension in the head,fidgetiness,irascibility and others as well as those of heart disorder, e.g., palpitation, insomnia and so on.

The heart controls the circulation of blood. The liver stores blood. Only when the blood of the heart is plentiful, does the liver have blood to store. When the blood of the liver is insufficient, the blood of the heart is certain to be deficient Therefore, signs and symptoms of a deficiency of the blood of the heart always occur in conjunction with an insufficiency of the blood of the liver. Many herbal medicines, such as Chinese angelica root (*Redix Angelicae Sinensis*), white peony root (*Radix Paeoniae Alba*), can nourish the blood of the liver and enrich the blood of the heart as well.

4) The Relationship between the Heart and the Kidney

The heart, with the property of *yang*, lies in the upper warmer and is classified as fire according to the theory of five elements. The kidney with the property of *yin*, lies in the lower warmer and is classified as water in light of the theory of

肢倦、面色少华等症，中医称之为“心脾两虚”，治疗常用健脾养心的归脾丸。

3）心与肝

心主神志，肝主疏泄，二者均与精神、情志活动有关，在病理上亦相互影响。如心阴不足、虚火内扰的患者，既可出现心烦、失眠、多梦等心病症状，又可兼见烦躁、易怒等肝病症状；肝阳上亢的患者，既为出现头晕、头胀、烦躁易怒等肝病症状，又可兼见心悸、失眠等心病症状。

心主血，肝藏血。心血充足，则肝有所藏；肝血不足，心血亦亏。所以心血不足与肝血不足的病症常同时并见。许多中药，如当归、白芍，既能补肝血，亦能补心血。

4）心与肾

心属阳，位于上，在五行属火；肾属阴，位于下，在五行属水。在正常生理情况下，心火必须下降于肾，以资肾阳，使肾水

five elements. When their physiological functions are normal, the fire of the heart is certain to descend into the kidney to nourish its *yang* (vital function) and warm its fluid. At the same time, the fluid of the kidney has to ascend into the heart to nourish the *yin* (vital essence) of the heart so that the *yang* (vital function) of the heart will not be excessive. The heart and the kidney have what is called in TCM an interdependent and interrestraining relationship characterized by mutual support and mutual check. When the *yang* of the heart is deficient and can not descent to warm the *yang* of the kidney an overflow of water due to a deficiency of the *yang* of the kidney occurs, which may attacks the heart, giving rise to palpitation, edema and the like. This is called "heart trouble caused by retention of water". When kidney fluid is insufficient and unable to ascend to nourish the *yin* (vital essence) of the heart, or when the *yang* (vital function) of the kidney is insufficient and unable to distill the *yin* (vital essence) of the kidney, the *yang* (vital function) of the heart will be excessive, such signs and symptoms as restlessness in mind, insomnia, dream-disturbed sleep and seminal emission will occur. And this is called "break-down of the normal physiological coordination between the heart and the kidney".

5) The Relationship between the Spleen and the Lung

The spleen has the function of transporting, distributing and transforming nutrients and promoting water metabolism, and is the source of nutrients for the growth and development of *qi* and blood. The lung performs the function of respiration and control the *qi* of the whole body. When the physiological functions are normal, the spleen can ensure that the lung works correctly by transporting food essence upward to nourish it; on the other hand, without the help of the lung in dispersing, descending and dredging, the spleen can not function well in transporting, distributing and transforming nutrients, or in

不寒；肾水亦必须上济于心，以资心阴，使心阳不亢。中医将心肾之间这种相互依存、相互制约的关系，称之为“心肾相交”。如心阳不振，不能下温肾阳，以致肾水不化，上凌于心，出现心悸、水肿等症，称之为“水气凌心”；若肾水不足，不能上滋心阴，或肾阳不足，不能蒸化肾阴，就会使心阳独亢，出现心烦、失眠、多梦、遗精等症，称之为“心肾不交”。

5）脾与肺

脾主运化，为气血生化之源；肺司呼吸，主人一身之气。在正常生理情况下，脾将水谷精微上输于肺，使肺得到营养，以保证其功能活动正常；另一方面，脾主运化水谷、水湿，亦有赖肺宣降、通调功能的协助。在病理情况下，脾气虚损，常可导致肺气不

promoting water metabolism. Pathologically, a deficiency and impairment of the *qi* (functional activities) of the spleen often leads to an insufficiency of the *qi* (functional activities) of the lung, which results in lassitude, shortness of breath and disinclination to talk. A dysfunction of the spleen in transportation and transformation causes an accumulation of fluid in the interior, which, in turn, leads to the formation of damp-phlegm. This will affect the lung's function of dispersing and descending *qi* and result in asthma, cough and excessive sputum. That is why it is said: "The spleen is the source of sputum, while the lung is the means to store it." A long-lasting lung disorder may also affect the function of the spleen. For example, when the *qi* (functional activities) of the lung is deficient and weak, the lung's function of dredging will be impaired, and fluid will accumulate in the interior. In this case, the *yang* (vital function) of the spleen will be stagnated, which results in edema, lassitude, distension of the abdomen and loose stools.

6) The Relationship between the Liver and the Lung

The lung lies in the upper warmer. Its *qi* (functional activities) disperses and descends, whereas the liver lies in the lower warmer, its *qi* (functional activities) disperses and ascends. Only when their *qi* (functional activities) ascends or descends properly, can it keep the movements of the *qi* of the whole body ascending and descending normally. The liver channel passes through the diaphragm and goes into the lung from the lower portion. When stagnant *qi* of the liver turns into fire and the fire sends its heat to the lung along the liver channel, the *yin* of the lung will be burned. This results in hypochondriac pain, irascibility, cough with dyspnea, hemoptysis and others. On the other hand, a dysfunction of the lung in dispersing and descending *qi* causes dryness and heat to go downward. This will impair the liver's function in smoothing and regulating the flow of vital energy and blood, and results in cough, moving

足，而见体倦乏力、少气懒言等症；脾失健运，水湿内停，聚为痰饮，影响肺的宣降，则可出现喘咳痰多等症，故有"脾为生痰之源，肺为贮痰之器"的说法。肺病日久，亦可影响脾的功能。如肺气虚衰，通调失职，水湿内停，可使脾阳受困，出现水肿、倦怠、腹胀、便溏等症。

6）肝与肺

肺居上焦，其气肃降；肝居下焦，其气升发。肝、肺升降得宜，才能维持人体气机的正常升降运动。肝的经脉由下而上贯膈注于肺，若肝郁化火，循经上逆，灼伤肺阴，可出现胁痛、易怒、咳逆、咯血等症，即"肝火犯肺"。相反，肺失肃降，燥热下行，

pains, distension and fullness in the sternocostal region, dizziness, headache and so on.

7) The Relationship between the Kidney and the Lung

The lung performs the function of respiration. The kidney has the function of controlling and promoting inspiration. The lung and the kidney coordinate to carry out the movement of respiration. The disorder of the above function of the kidney due to a deficiency of its *qi* or affected by a prolonged deficiency of the *qi* of the lung is the cause of inspiratory dyspnea which is worse in movement.

The lung is the upper source of the circulation of water. Only by the lung's functions of activating the flow of vital energy, blood and body fluid, and cleaning inspired air and keeping it flowing downwards, can food essence in the upper part of the body cavity be distributed to all parts of the body, and the fluid produced after metabolism be carried downwards into the kidney and then into the urinary bladder. The kidney has the function of dominating water metabolism. Only by this function can water coming into the kidney from the upper part of the body be divided into clear and turbid fluids. Clear fluid flows back throughout the body by way of the triple warmer. Turbid fluid is turned into urine and carried into the urinary bladder. A dysfunction of the lung in activating and dredging the flow of vital energy and body fluid, and a dysfunction of the kidney in dominating water metabolism can affect normal water metabolism. Not only that, the two often affect each other, resulting in severe disturbance of water metabolism, which is indicated by a very severe cough and asthmatic breathing when going to sleep, edema and so on.

Also, the *yin* (vital essence) of the lung and the kidney nourish each other. A long-term deficiency of the *yin* (vital essence) of the lung may damage the *yin* (vital essence) of the kidney. A deficiency and impairment of the *yin* (vital essence)

亦可影响肝的疏泄功能，出现咳嗽、胸胁引痛胀满、头晕、头痛等症。

7）肾与肺

肺司呼吸，肾主纳气。肺、肾相互配合，共同完成呼吸运动。若肾气不足，摄纳无权；或肺气久虚，穷必及肾，以致肾不纳气，均可出现呼多吸少、动则尤甚等症。

肺为水上之源，只有通过肺的宣发、肃降，才能使在上之水谷精微布散全身，代谢后的水液下归于肾，输入膀胱；肾有气化水液的功能，下归肾脏的水液，只有通过肾的气化作用，才能使清者升腾，通过三焦，回流体内；浊者化为尿液，输入膀胱。如肺的宣降、通调功能失职，或肾的气化不利，不仅都可影响水液的正常代谢，而且二者之间又常互相影响，造成严重的水液代谢障碍，出现咳逆喘息不得卧、水肿等。

此外，肺、肾之阴液亦互相滋养。若肺阴久虚，可损及肾阴；

of the kidney may also lead to an insufficiency of the *yin* (vital essence) of the lung. In either case, a deficiency of the *yin* (vital essence) of both the lung and the kidney will be indicated by dry cough, hoarse voice, malar flush, tidal fever, night sweating, lassitude of loins and legs. On treating these, the *yin* (vital essence) of the lung and the kidney are often replenished together.

8) The Relationship between the Liver and the Spleen

The liver has the function of smoothing and regulating the flow of vital energy and blood, while the spleen has the function of transporting, distributing and transforming nutrients, and promoting water metabolism. When this function of the liver is normal, then the spleen's function of sending food essence upward and keeping *qi* (vital energy) moving upward and the stomach's function of sending down food content are both moderate and normal and the spleen functions well in transporting and distributing nutrients and water. This ensures a plentiful source of food essence which is carried continuously to the liver. Thus the liver is nourished and functions well in smoothing and regulating the flow of vital energy and blood. The disorder of the above functions of the liver may affect the functions of the spleen and the stomach, resulting in the syndrome of "incoordination between the liver and the spleen (stomach), marked by a feeling of fullness in the chest and hypochondria, poor appetite, abdominal distension after eating, belching and discomfort, abdominal pain, diarrhea and so on. On the other hand, a disorder of the spleen may also affect the liver. For example ,a dysfunction of the spleen in transporting and distributing nutrients and water will lead to an insufficient source of vital energy and blood, which leads to malnourishment of the liver and resulsts in the syndrome of deficiency of blood of the liver. The heat engendered by dampness accumulated in the spleen impairs the liver and the gallbladder's function of smoothing and regulating the

肾阴亏损，亦可致肺阴不足。二者均可出现干咳、音哑、颧红、潮热、盗汗、腰膝酸软等肺肾阴虚的病症。治疗时常同补肺、肾之阴。

8）肝与脾

肝主疏泄，脾主运化。肝的疏泄功能正常，则脾胃升降适度，运化健全；脾气健运，水谷精微化源充足，不断地输送、滋养于肝，肝才能得以发挥正常的疏泄作用。如肝失疏泄，影响脾胃的升降、运化，可形成“肝脾(胃)不和”的证候，表现为胸胁满闷、食欲不振、食后腹胀、嗳气不舒、腹痛泄泻等。反之，脾病亦可影响于肝。如脾失健运，气血化源不足，肝失所养，可形成肝血不足；脾不化湿，郁而化热，影响肝胆疏泄，胆汁外溢肌肤，可

flow of vital energy and blood and causes bile to overflow to the skin causing jaundice.

9) The Relationship between the Spleen and the Kidney

The spleen transports and transforms food essence and provides the material basis for the acquired constitution. The kidney stores the essence of life (either congenital or acquired), control the fire of the "vital gate", and is the foundation of the native constitution. The spleen can only function well in transportation and transformation when warmed by the *yang* (vital function) of the kidney (which is believed to be the source of heat energy of the body). The essence of life stored in the kidney can only be plentiful when provided continuously with the food essence transformed by the spleen. The spleen and the kidney subsidize and promote each other and also affect each other pathologically. For example, when the *yang* (vital function) of the kidney is too deficient to warm the *yang* (vital function) of the spleen, or when a long-term deficiency of the *yang* (vital function) of the spleen involves the *yang* (vital function) of the kidney, the syndrome of the deficiency of the *yang* (vital functin) of both the spleen and the kidney will, in the end, occur marked by morning diarrhea, watery stools mixed with undigested food, and cold and painful sensation in the abdomen.

In addition, the spleen transports and transforms water and dampness, the kidney regulates water circulation and helps maintain the fluid balance of the body. They both coordinate to play an important role in promoting water metabolism. When they fail to perform this function, coldness of the body and limbs, difficulty in urinating and edema occur, which in TCM, is called "an overflow of water (edema) due to a deficiency of *yang* (vital function)". In the treatment, *Zhen Wu* Decoction is often presceibe which has the efficacy of warming and recuperating the *yang* of the spleen and kidney and promoting diuresis.

出现黄疸。

9）脾与肾

脾主运化水谷精微，为后天之本；肾主藏精，寓命门真火，为先天之本。脾的运化，必得肾中阳气的温煦，始能健运；肾脏精气，又有赖于脾所化生之水谷精微的不断补充，才能充盛。二者相互资助，相互促进。在病理上亦互相影响，如肾阳不足，不能温煦脾阳；或脾阳久虚，损及肾阳，最终均可致成五更泄泻、下利清谷、腹部冷痛之脾肾阳虚证。

此外，脾主运化水湿，肾能气化水液，二者相互配合，在水液代谢中发挥重要作用。如脾肾阳虚，不能化水，可出现形寒肢冷、小便不利、水肿等，中医称之为“阳虚水泛”。治疗常用温阳（温补脾肾阳气）利水之真武汤。

10) The Relationship between the Liver and the Kidney

The liver stores blood, and the kidney stores the essence of life. The blood of the liver depends on nourishment from the essence of life in the kidney, while the essence of life stored in the kidney depends on replenishment from the blood of the liver. Because TCM believes that blood can develop into the essence of life, and vice versa, and their source is the same food essence, it is said, "The essence of life and blood have a common source." and "The liver and the kidneys have a common source." Pathologically, a deficiency of the essence of life in the kidney may lead to a dificiency of the blood of the liver. A long-term deficiency of the blood of the liver may also cause a deficiency of the essence of life in the kidney. Therefore, in treating the deficiency of the *yin* of the liver or kidneys, a method is often used to reinforce the *yin* of both the liver and kidney.

2. The Relationship between Viscera and Bowels

Viscera belong to *yin* ,whereas bowels belong to *yang*. Viscera are considered as being interior, whereas bowels are exterior. The exterior and interior relationship between a viscus and a bowel is formed by the connections between their channels. They not only act in coordination with each other physiologically but also affect each other pathologically .

1) The Relationship between the Heart and the Small Intestine

The Channel of Hand-*Shaoyin* belongs to the heart and connects with the small intestine downward, whereas the Channel of Hand-*Taiyang* belongs to the small intestine and connects with the heart upward, thus forming an exterior and interior relationship between the heart and the small intestine. This

10）肝与肾

肝藏血，肾藏精。肝血有赖于肾精的滋养，肾精又有赖于肝血的补充。由于中医认可精血可以互生，其化源均来之水谷精微，故有"精血同源"、"肝肾同源"的说法。在病理上，肾精亏损，可致肝血（阴）不足；肝血（阴）久虚，亦可导致肾精亏损。因此，在治疗肝阴虚或肾阴虚时，常用肝、肾同补法。

2. 脏与腑的关系

脏属阴，腑属阳；脏为里，腑为表。脏与腑通过其经脉互相络属，构成表里关系。它们在生理上互相配合，在病理上亦相互影响。

1）心与小肠

心手少阴之脉属心，下络小肠；小肠手太阳之脉属小肠，上络于心，二者构成表里关系。心与小肠的内在联系，表现在病理

relationship is obvious pathologically. For example, the accumulated heat in the heart can move to the small intestine, causing pathogenic heat to collect in the small intestine manifested as deep-colored urine, oliguria and burning pains in urination. The excessive heat in the small intestine may also go upward along the Channel of Hand-*Taiyang* to burn the heart, causing the fire of the heart to flare up and lead to mental irritability and ulcers in the mouth and on the tongue. In treating these two syndromes, Powder Treating Dark Urine is often prescribed. Its functions are to clear away heart-fire and promote diuresis.

2) The Relationship between the Lung and the Large Intestine

The exterior and interior relationship between the lung and the large intestine is formed by connections of their channels. As the *qi* (functional activities) of the lung cleanses inspired air and keeps it flowing downward, the *qi* of the large intestine descends and maintains normal transportation, so that feces are excreted freely. The normal functioning of the large intestine in transportation, on the other hand, benefits the free movement of the *qi* of the bowels and the descent of the *qi* of the lung. Pathologically, a dysfunction of the lung in sending down its *qi* prevents the body fluid from descending and affects the function of the large intestine in transportation so as to cause difficulty in defecating. Constipation and the stoppage of the *qi* of the bowels may also affect the descent of the *qi* of the lung, causing asthmatic cough and distension in the chest. Drugs which disperse and lower the *qi* of the lung and nourish and moisten the *yin* of the lung are often taken into consideration in the treatment of constipation. For example, root of balloonflower (*Radix Platycodi*), apricot kernel (*Semen Amarum Armeniace*) and the like are prescribed. In the treatment of dyspnea due the stasis of lung-*qi*, the drugs which relax the bowels often come into the doctor's mind.

上较为明显。如心经有热，可移热小肠，出现尿赤。尿少、尿道灼痛等小肠实热的病症；小肠有热，亦可循经上熏于心，出现心烦、口舌生疮等心火内炽的病症。治疗均可采用清心利尿的导赤散。

2）肺与大肠

肺与大肠亦通过其经脉的相互络属构成表里关系。肺气肃降，则大肠之气随之而降，传导功能正常，大便排出通畅；而大肠传导正常，腑气通畅，亦有利于肺气的肃降。在病理上，肺失肃降，津液不能下达，可影响大肠的传导功能而大便困难；大便秘结，腑气不通，又可影响肺气的肃降而喘咳胸闷。在治疗上，大便秘结常酌加桔梗、杏仁等宣降肺气、滋润肺阴之药；肺闭实喘，有时亦酌用通利大便之品。

3) The Relationship between the Spleen and the Stomach

Both the spleen and the stomach lie in the middle warmer. Their channels connect them to each other and form their exterior and interior relationship. The stomach receives food, while the spleen transports, distributes and transforms nutrients Moreover, the spleen helps the stomach with digestion and fluid transportation. It is appropriate for the *qi* of the stomach to descend, and for the *qi* of the spleen to ascend. The stomach likes moisture but hates dryness. The spleen likes dryness but hates dampness. They both share the work and coordinate to fulfil the task of digesting and absorbing food, and transporting and transforming food essence by the ascent of one and the descent of the other, the moisture of one and the dryness of the other. Pathologically, they affect each other. For example, a deficiency of *yang* and a presence of cold in the spleen is often accompanied by an insufficiency of *yang* of the stomach, which is called "a deficiency and cold of the middle warmer." In the treatment, the spleen and the stomach should be treated together, and the method of warming the middle warmer and dispelling the cold can be used.

4) The Relationship between the Liver and the Gallbladder

The liver and the gallbladder are connected by their channels to form their exterior and interior relationship. The liver has the function of smoothing and regulating the flow of vital energy and blood. Its surplus vital energy helps to form bile. The gallbladder is located under the liver and in charge of the storage and excretion of bile. Only when the liver functions normally in smoothing and regulating the flow of vital energy and blood can bile be secreted, stored and excreted normally. On the other hand only when bile is excreted without any obstruction can the liver give full play to its dredging function. Pathologically, liver diseases often involve the gallbladder and gallbladder diseases often involve the liver as

3）脾与胃

脾胃同居中焦，有经脉互相络属，构成表里关系。胃主受纳，脾主运化，脾为胃行其津液；胃气宜降，脾气宜升；胃喜润恶燥，脾喜燥恶湿，二者一升一降，一润一燥，分工合作，共同完成饮食物的消化、吸收与水谷精微的转输。在病理上，二者亦互相影响。如脾脏虚寒，常同时兼有胃阳不足，中医常称之为“中焦虚寒”，治疗亦脾胃同治，如温中散寒法。

4）肝与胆

肝与胆有经脉互相络属，构成表里关系。肝主疏泄，其余气生成胆汁。胆附于肝，主胆汁的贮存、排泄。肝的疏泄功能正常，胆汁才能正常地分泌、贮藏和排泄；胆汁排泄无阻，肝才能发挥其疏泄功能。在病理上，肝病常影响及胆，胆病亦常累及到肝，

well. As a result they both suffer. For example, the liver and the gallbladder may, at the same time, suffer from stagnation of vital energy and heat or dampness and heat. In this case, the liver and the gallbladder should be treated together. This may include "removing the stagnation of vital energy of both the liver and the gallbladder" and "clearing away the dampness and heat from both the liver and the gallbladder".

5) The Relationship between the Kidney and the Urinary Bladder

The kidney and the urinary bladder are connected by their channels to form their exterior and interior relationship. The kidney is a viscus that serves to control water and to maintain fluid balance by excreting or retaining the water in the body. The urinary bladder is a bowel which serves to store and excrete urine. Whether the functions of the urinary bladder are normal is closely related to whether vital energy of the kidney is sufficient. When the vital energy of the kidney is sufficient, the kidney regulates properly the excretion and retention of water, resulting in the normal functioning of the urinary bladder in storing and excreting urine. When the vital energy of the kidney is deficient, the urinary bladder will lose its power to control urine, causing incontinence of urine or enuresis. If there is a deficiency of the vital energy, the kidney will fail to effectively regulate water metabolism, which obstructs the urinary bladder in the excretion of urine. In this instance difficulty in urination or urodialysis will occur. Treatment often begins by reinforcing the vital energy or the essence of the kidney.

3. The Relationship between Bowels

The chief functions of the six bowels are to transport and transform water and food. Therefore, their relations are shown mainly in the process of digesting and absorbing food and excreting waste.

终则肝胆同病，如肝胆郁热、肝胆湿热等。治疗则肝胆同治，如疏肝利胆、清利肝胆湿热等治法。

5）肾与膀胱

肾与膀胱有经脉互相络属，配为表里关系。肾司开阖，为主水之脏。膀胱主贮存、排泄尿液，为主水之腑。膀胱的功能正常与否与肾气的盛衰密切相关。肾气充足，开阖有度，则膀胱贮尿排尿的功能正常。如肾气不足，膀胱固摄无权，可见小便失禁或遗尿；肾虚气化无力，膀胱排泄障碍，则见小便不利或尿闭。治疗多从补肾入手。

3．腑与腑的关系

六腑的主要功能是传化水谷。它们之间的关系因而主要体现在饮食物的消化、吸收和排泄过程中。

Food arriving in the stomach is turned into chyme after it has been ground, fermented and disgested by the stomach and spleen. Chyme passes to the small intestine. The small intestine receives and further digests the chyme. At the same time, the gallbladder excretes bile into the small intestine to aid in digestion. The chyme is fully digested in the small intestine and then changes into two parts, the useful (clarity) and the waste (turbidity). "Clarity" is food essence and is transported and distributed to all parts of the body by the spleen. "Turbidity" is the waste of water and food. The waste water goes into the kidney, then to the urinary bladder. There it is turned into urine to be excreted from the body. Food waste passes into the large intestine, changes into feces and leaves the body via the anus. In the above process of transportation and transformation of water and food, the combined functional activities of triple warmer take part. While the six bowels transport and transform water and food, the process of receiving, digesting, transporting and excreting continues. Any of the bowels may be hollow one moment and full the next. So it is appropriate for them to be kept clear and free from obstruction. This is why there is theory in TCM such as "The six bowels function well when unobstructed". Pathologically, disorders among the six blowels often affect each other. For instance, when body fluid is consumed because of excessive heat in the stomach, the large intestine will have trouble in transportation, and constipation will occur. A disturbance of the large intestine in transmission and transformation not only leads to obstruction of vital energy of the large intestine, but also affects the regular descent of that of the stomach, causing repeated vomiting. A dominant gallbladder fire often interferes with the stomach and causes vomiting of bitter fluid. Dampness and heat accumulated in the stomach and spleen suffocate and steam the liver and the gallbladder. This may cause bile to overflow, and give rise to jaundice.

饮食入胃，经过胃的腐熟、脾的消磨，变成食糜，下降于小肠。小肠承受由胃而来的食糜，做进一步的消化；同时，胆排泄胆汁进入小肠，以协助消化。食糜在小肠内被充分消化、泌别清浊后，其清者为水谷精微，由脾转输全身；其浊者为水谷糟粕，其中的水液经肾入膀胱，变为尿液，排出体外；食物残渣则进入大肠，变为粪便，由肛门排出。当然，在上述传化水谷的过程中，还有三焦的气化作用。由于六腑传化水谷，需要不断地受纳、消化、传导和排泄，更虚更实，宜通不宜滞，故中医有“六腑以通为用”的理论。在病理上，六腑之间常互相影响，互相传变。如胃有实热，消烁津液，可致大肠传导障碍，出现大便秘结；大肠传导障碍，腑气不通又可影响胃气和降而症见呕吐频作；胆火炽盛，常有犯胃，出现呕吐苦水；脾胃湿热，熏蒸肝胆，胆汁外溢，又可发为黄疸。

Modern medical men have been treating acute abdomen such as cholelithiasis, intestinal obstruction and appendicitis by "removing the stagnation of the gallbladder to discharge the stone", "administering laxatives and purgatives for removing stagnation of food and water and restoring normal bowel movement" and "dispersing blood stasis and dredging collateral". The curative effects of these are very good. All these methods are based on the physiological characteristic of the bowels — the hollowness following fullness of the bowels without end. The six bowels, of course, may also suffer from a deficiency syndrome and a cold syndrome. In clinical practice they should be treated according to their specific pathogenesis.

近代医家根据六腑更虚更实的生理特点，采用利胆排石、通里攻下、化瘀行滞等法治疗胆结石、肠梗阻、阑尾炎等急腹症，效果甚佳。当然，六腑亦有虚证、寒证，临床上应辨明病机，随证治之。

Chapter Four

The Theory of *Qi*, Blood and Body Fluid

TCM believes that the *qi* ,blood and body fluid are the basic components of the body and maintain the life activities of the human body. It is from *qi*, blood and body fluid that comes the energy needed by viscera and bowels, channels and collaterals, tissues and other organs for performing their physiological functions. On the other hand, their formation and metabolism depend on the normal physiological functions of viscera and bowels, channels and collaterals, tissues and other organs. Therefore, it is true to say that *qi*, blood and body fluid are not only the material basis of the functional activities of viscera and bowels, channels and collaterals, tissues and other organs, but also the physiological products of their functional activities. They complement each other and have mutual causality in many aspects such as physiology and pathology.

The theory of *qi*, blood and body fluid is a theory used to study the development, transportation and distribution, physiological functions, pathological changes and mutual relations of *qi*, blood and body fluid of the human body.

Section 1

Qi

1. The Concept of *Qi*

What is meant by *qi* ? The concept of *qi* is based on the ancient Chinese initial undertanding of natural phenomena.

第 四 章

气血津液学说

中医学认为，气、血、津液是构成人体和维持人体生命活动的基本物质。人体脏腑、经络、组织、器官进行生理活动所需要的能量来源于气血津液，而气血津液的生成与代谢，又依赖于脏腑、经络、组织、器官的正常生理活动。因此，可以认为，气血津液既是脏腑、经络、组织、器官功能活动的物质基础，又是其功能活动的生理产物。它们在生理、病理诸方面，都是相辅相成，互为因果的。

气血津液学说，就是研究人体气、血、津液的生成、输布、生理功能、病理变化及其相互关系的学说。

第一节　气

1. 气的概念

何谓气？气是古代人们对自然现象的一种朴素认识，即认为

That is, *qi* is the most basic substance of which the world is comprised. Everything in the universe results from the movements and changes of *qi*. This concept was introduced into TCM and became one of its characteristics. After a comprehensive survey of the statements on *qi* in TCM documents, we have come to the conclusion that the meaning of *qi* in TCM has two aspects. One refers to the vital substances comprising the human body and maintaining its life activities, such as the *qi* of water and food (food essence), the *qi* of breathing (breathing nutrients) and so on. The other refers to the physiological functions of viscera and bowels, channels and collaterals, such as the *qi* of the heart, the lung, the spleen and the stomach and so on. The *qi* here referred to, is specifically the physiological functions of these viscera and bowels.

2. The Formation of *Qi*

The *qi* in the human body is different in classification and formation. But, generally speaking, it has no more than two sources. One is the innate vital substance one inherits from one's parents before birth. The other is the food essence and fresh air one receives from air, water and food in the natural world. The materials obtained in the two ways above have to be processed and tranformed by the viscera and bowels before becoming the *qi* of the human body. The process for *qi* to be formed is as follows :The innate vital substance acted on by the kidney comes out of the gate of life (the portion between the two kidneys) and goes up to the middle warmer. There it combines with the food essence coming from the spleen and continues upwards until it combines with the fresh air inhaled by the lung. Finally it turns into *qi*. It is easy to see from the above that the *qi* of the human body is formed through the joint work of the kidney, the spleen ,the stomach and the lung in combining the innate vital substance taken from one's parents, the food essence received from water and food, and

气是构成世界的最基本物质，宇宙间的一切事物，都是气运动变化的结果。这种观点被引入中医领域，逐渐形成了中医特有的“气”概念。纵观中医文献中有关气的论述，其含义有二：一是指构成人体和维持人体生命活动的精微物质，如水谷之气、呼吸之气等；二是指脏腑、经络的生理功能，如心气、肺气、脾气、胃气等，即特指这些脏腑的生理功能。

2. 气的生成

人体之气，种类非一，生成各异。但从总体上说，其资生之源不外以下两个方面：即出生之前从父母禀受的先天之精气，出生之后从自然界获得的水谷之精气和清气。从以上两个途径获得的“原料”，还须通过人体多个脏腑的加工、转化，才能生成具有生命力的人体之气。其生成过程是：先天之精气在肾的作用下，出肾间(命门)，向上至中焦，与脾胃化生的水谷之精气相并；继续向上，与肺吸入的清气相合。最后，生成了具有生命力的“气”。由上不难看出，人体之气是通过肾、脾胃、肺等脏腑的综合作用，

the fresh air obtained from nature.

3. The Functions of Qi

Different kinds of *qi* have different functions. Generally speaking, they can be summarized as follows:

1) Promoting Action

Qi is a sort of essence full of vitality. It can help activate the growth and development of the human body, promote the physiological functions of each viscus, bowel, channel, collateral, tissue and organ and speed up the formation and circulation of blood and the metabolism of body fluid as well. For example, if the above functions are weakened as a result of the deficiency of *qi* (vital energy), the following will occur: late and slow growth and development of the human body or senilism; weakened functions of viscera and bowels, channels and collaterals, tissues and other organs; insufficient blood formation or stagnation in blood vessels; and disturbance in the metabolism of body fluid.

2) Warming Action

Nan Jing (***Classic on Medical Problems***) says: "*Qi* has a warming action." *Qi* is the main source of the heat needed by the human body. The body keeps its constant temperature mainly through the warming action of its *qi*. A deficiency of *qi* can cause lowered body temperature, intolerance to cold and cold limbs.

3) Defending Action

The defending action of *qi* is shown in two aspects. One is to guard the surface of the skin against the exopathogen. The other is to combat the invading exopathogen so as to ward it off. When the defending function of *qi* is normal, the exopathogen has difficulty in invading the body, even though

将先天之精气、水谷之精气和自然界之气结合而成的。

3. 气的功能

不同的气，有其不同的功能。概而言之，可归纳如下：

1）推动作用

气是活力很强的精微物质，它能激发人体的生长、发育，推动各脏腑、经络、组织、器官的生理功能，推动血的生成与循行以及津液的代谢。如气虚而上述功能减弱，则会出现人体生长、发育迟缓或早衰，脏腑、经络、组织、器官功能减弱，血的生成不足或血脉瘀滞，以及津液代谢障碍等。

2）温煦作用

《难经》说："气主煦之。"气是人体热量的重要来源，人体所以能保持恒定的体温，主要依赖气的温煦作用。如果气的温煦作用减弱，就会出现体温下降、畏寒怯冷、四肢不温等虚寒病症。

3）防御作用

气的防御作用包括两个方面：一是护卫肌表，防御外邪入侵；二是与侵入人体的病邪相争，以驱邪外出。气的防御功能正常，

it may obtain entry, it is not certain to cause any disease. If it does cause a disease, this disease is easy to cure. When the defending function of *qi* becomes weaker, when the ability of the human body to fight the exopathogen is lowered, the body is easily invaded and diseases are caused. And what is more, these diseases are hard to cure.

4) Consolidating and Governing Action

By "consolidating and governing action", we mean that *qi* has the ability to command, control and consolidate the liquid substances and organs in the abdominal cavity. This is done by:

(1) Keeping the blood flowing within, not extravasating out of, the vessels;

(2) Controlling and adjusting the secretion and excretion of sweat, urine and saliva, and preventing the body fluid from escaping;

(3) Consolidating and storing sperm and preventing emission and premature ejaculation;

(4) Consolidating the organs so as to prevent them from descending.

A decrease in the above functions of *qi* may cause various kinds of hemorrhage, spontaneous perspiration, polyuria, salivation, spermatorrhea, premature ejaculation, prolapse of the stomach, kidney and uterus.

The consolidating and governing action and the promoting action of *qi* oppose each other and yet also complement each other. On the one hand, *qi* has the function of promoting the circulation of blood, and the transportation and distribution of body fluid. On the other hand, it also has the function of controlling and adjusting the movement, secretion and excretion of liquid substances in the body. The coordination and balance of these two functions are essential for maintaining normal blood circulation and water metabolism within the body.

则外邪不易侵入；即使侵入，也不一定发病；就是发病，也容易痊愈。如果气的防御功能减弱，人体抵御外邪的能力降低，一方面机体易被外邪侵袭而发病；另一方面，患病后也难以很快痊愈。

4）固摄作用

所谓固摄，乃指气对体内的液态物质和腹腔脏器等具有统摄、控制和固定作用，主要体现在以下几个方面：

（1）统摄血液在脉管内正常循行而不外溢；

（2）控制、调节汗液、尿液、唾液等的分泌、排泄，防止体液丢失；

（3）固藏精液，防止遗泄；

（4）固定脏器位置，防止下移。

如果气的以上功能减退，可引起各种出血、自汗、多尿、流涎、遗精、早泄以及胃、肾、子宫等脏器下垂。

气的固摄作用与推动作用是相反相成的。一方面，气能推动血液循行和津液输布；另一方面，气又能控制、调节体内液态物质的运行、分泌与排泄。这两方面作用的协调、平衡，是维持人体正常血液循行和津液代谢的必要条件。

5) Promoting Metabolism and Transformation

"*Qi hua*" is a specific term in the science of TCM. It refers, in general, to various kinds of changes taking place in the body under the action of *qi*. Specifically, it refers to the metabolism of fundamental substances, vital energy, blood and body fluid, and the transformations which can occur between them. For example, vital energy, blood and body fluid are formed in the following manner: ingested food is changed into food essence, and food essence is, in turn, transformed into vital energy, blood or body fluid, and these can then be changed into any one of the others according to the physiological need of the body. The waste from the eaten food and the products produced in the course of metabolism are changed, separately, into feces, urine and sweat which are ready to be removed from the body. All these are the specific manifestations of the action of the activity of *qi*. The dysfunction of *qi* in performing its action will affect the whole metabolism of the body. That is to say, it will affect the digestion, absorption, transformation and transportation of food: the formation, movement and transformation of vital energy, blood and body fluid; and the excretion of feces, urine and sweat; thus causing varous symptoms associated with abnormal metabolism. In short, the process in which *qi* performs its functions is the process in which the substances in the body are metabolized, and in which the substances and energy are transformed.

Although the above five functions of *qi* are different, they enjoy close cooperation and mutual support.

4. The Movement of *Qi*

The various functions of *qi* are all performed by its movement. TCM calls the movement of *qi* as "functional activities of *qi*". Different types of *qi* move in different ways. Theoretically, however, we can put them in four basic ways: ascending,

5）气化作用

气化，是中医学特有的一个术语，泛指在气的作用下体内所发生的各种变化。具体地说，是指精、气、血、津液各自的新陈代谢及其相互转化。例如：气、血、津液的生成，都需要将饮食物转化成水谷精微，然后再化生为气、血、津液等；它们还可根据机体的生理需要而相互转化；饮食物的残渣与机体代谢后的产物，则分别转化成粪便、尿液和汗液等，排出体外。这些都是气化作用的具体体现。如果气化失职，则能影响整个人体的物质代谢，如饮食物的消化、吸收与转输，气、血、津液的生成、运行与转化，以及粪便、尿液和汗液等的排泄，从而形成各种代谢异常的病证。所以说，气化的过程，就是体内物质代谢的过程，是物质转化和能量转化的过程。

气的以上五个功能，虽各不相同，但又都是密切配合、相互为用的。

4. 气的运动

气的各种功能，是通过气的运动来实现的。中医将气的运动，称为“气机”。不同的气，有其不同的运动形式。但从理论上，可

descending, exiting and entering. Ascending refers to the movement from below; descending, from above; exiting, from the interior; and entering from the exterior. These movements of *qi* are vital to life. Once they stop, life comes to an end.

They are not only seen in promoting and activating various kinds of physiological activities in the human body, but also seen in motivating the physiological activities of the viscera and bowels, channels and collaterals, tissues and other organs. For example, while the lung performs its function, exhaling is exiting, inhaling is entering, dispersing is ascending and keeping the inspired air flowing downward is descending. Of course, this doesn't mean each organ functions in all four types of movement. Some organs only function in a particular one. For instance, it is appropriate for the *qi* of the spleen to ascend and the *qi* of the stomach to descend. However, in view of all the physiological activities of the body, the four movements of *qi* have to be coordinated and balanced. Only in this way can the physiological functions of the human body remain normal.

In TCM, the physiological state in which the four basic movements of *qi* are coordinated and balanced is called "harmonious functional activities of *qi*". When they are uncoordinated and unbalanced it is called "disharmonious functional activities of *qi*". Because the movements of *qi* differ, the disharmonious funcitonal activities of *qi* are shown in various ways. For example, over-ascending is known as "the abnormal rising of *qi*"; not descending on time, "the non-descending of *qi*"; not ascending on time or over-descending, "the sinking of *qi*". Exiting too much because it is unable to be contained is known as "the escape of *qi*", while an accumulation inside due to its being unable to exit is known as "the accumulation of *qi*" or "depressed *qi*", and even "closed *qi*" when the accumulation is more severe. If *qi* has difficulty in moving or its flow is even partially obstructed it is called "the stagnation of *qi*".

将其归纳为升、降、出、入四种基本运动形式。升，是指气由下而上的运动；降，乃指气由上而下的运动；出，是指气由体内向体外的运动；入，则指气由体外向体内的运动。气的升降出入是人体生命活动的一种表现，升降出入一旦停止，人的生命也就终止了。

气的升降出入，不仅推动、激发人体的各种生理活动，而且具体体现于脏腑、经络、组织、器官的生理活动之中。如肺的呼吸功能，呼气为出，吸气为入，宣发为升，肃降为降。当然，并不是每一脏器的功能，都包括升、降、出、入，而是有所侧重。如脾气宜升，胃气宜降等。但就整个机体的生理活动来看，升与降，出与入，必须保持协调、平衡，才能维持人体正常的生理功能。

中医把气的升、降、出、入运动协调、平衡的生理状态，称之为“气机调畅”；把升、降、出、入失去协调、平衡，称为“气机失调”。由于气的运动形式不一，所以气机失调的表现形式也多种多样。如气上升太过，为“气逆”；气下降不及，为“气不降”；气上升不及或下降太过，为“气陷”；气不能内守而外出太过，为“气脱”；气不能外达而结聚于内，为“气结”或“气郁”，甚则“气

As to individual internal organs, the examples of the disharmonious functional activities of *qi* are as follows :the non-descending of the *qi* of the lung, the sinking of the *qi* of the spleen, the adverse rising of the *qi* of the stomach, the nonconsolidation of the *qi* of the kidney, etc.

5. The Classification of *Qi*

The *qi* of the human body is classified into the following categories:

1) Inborn *Qi*

Yuan Qi

Inborn *qi* is also called "primordial *qi*" or "genuine *qi*". It is the most important and fundamental of all.

(1) Formation

Inborn *qi* comes mainly from the innate essence stored in the kidney. But it also depends on the supplement and nourishment of the acquired essence developed in the spleen and stomach. This is what The Acupuncture Therapy And The Relation Between Healthy Energy And Pathogen, a chapter of ***Miraculous Pivot***, says: "The inborn *qi* is received from heaven and combined with food essence to nourish the body."

(2) Movement

The inborn *qi* commences from "the vital gate", the portion between the two kidneys, passes the triple warmer and circulates throughout the body. It goes inward to the five viscera and six bowels and outward to the muscles and skin, i.e., the superficial layer of the body. It goes everywhere and acts on all parts of the body.

(3) Functions

The inborn *qi* has the functions of both activating growth and development and promoting the functional activities of all the viscera and bowels, channels and collaterals, tissues and other organs. Therefore, the inborn *qi* is the motivating power

闭”；气的运行受阻，甚至局部阻滞不通，为“气滞”。就某一脏腑而言，如肺气不降、脾气下陷、胃气上逆、肾不纳气等。

5. 气的分类

人体之气可分为以下数种：

1）元气

元气，又名“原气”、“真气”，是人体各种气中最重要、最基本的一种。

（1）生成

元气主要由肾所藏的先天之精气所化生，又赖脾胃化生的后天之精所充养。此即《灵枢·刺节真邪》所说：“真气者，所受于天，与谷气并而充身者也。”

（2）运行

元气发于肾间（命门），通过三焦循行全身，内至五脏六腑，外达肌肤腠理，无处不到，以作用于机体的各个部分。

（3）功能

元气有激发人体的生长、发育和推动各脏腑、经络、组织、器官功能活动的作用。所以说，元气是人体生命活动的原动力。

of the vital activities of the human body. Sufficient inborn *qi* causes normal growth and development of the body and healthy and vigorous activities of all the functions of the body. Insufficient inborn *qi* leads to late and slow growth and development, and reduces all physiological functions. This is indicated by lassitude, general debility and susceptibility to diseases.

2) Pectoral *Qi*

Pectoral *qi* is the *qi* stored in the chest.

(1) Formation

Pectoral *qi* is a combination of the fresh air inhaled by the lung and the food essence derived by the spleen and stomach from water and grain.

(2) Movement

Pectoral *qi* is stored in the chest and poured into the channels of the heart and lung just as Five Kinds of Flavour, a chapter of ***Miraculous Pivot***, says: "It goes out of the lung and circulates through the larynx and pharynx. This is the reason why it exits when being exhaled and enters when being inhaled." The book ***Classified Canon*** compiled by Zhang Jiebin in 1624 A.D. says: "It goes down to the elixir field to be stored, and fills the Point Qijie of the *Yangming* Channel from which it continues to go downward to the feet."

(3) Functions

Pectoral *qi*, in the main, has two functions. One is that it flows through the respiratory tract to promote the respiratory movement of the lung and is involved in the loudness or softness of vioce and words. The other is that it fills the heart channel to promote and adjust its beat, and to promote and adjust the circulation of blood and vital energy. It also exerts an influence on the warmth and activities of the limbs. Therefore, the manifestations of a deficiency of pectoral *qi* are, often, the weakness of the functions of the heart and lung, such as

元气充足，则人体生长、发育正常，各种功能活动健旺；元气不足，则生长、发育迟缓，各种生理功能衰退，表现为神疲乏力、体弱多病等。

2）宗气

宗气，乃指积于胸中之气。

（1）生成

宗气是由肺从自然界吸入的清气和脾胃从饮食物中化生的水谷精气结合而成。

（2）运行

宗气聚集于胸中，贯注于心肺之脉，上"出于肺，循喉咽，故呼则出，吸则入"（见《灵枢·五味》）；下"蓄于丹田，注足阳明之气街而下行至足"（见《类经》）。

（3）功能

宗气的功能主要有两个方面：一是走息道以促进肺的呼吸运动，并与语言、声音的强弱有关；二是贯心脉以推动、调节心脏的搏动以及血气的运行，并影响着肢体的寒温与活动。故宗气不足，多表现为心、肺功能衰弱，如呼吸微弱、语声低微、心动异常、血行缓慢、肢体厥冷、倦怠乏力和运动不灵等。在临床上，

shallow breathing, soft voice, abnormal heartbeat, slow blood flow, cold limbs, lassitude and moving with difficulties. In clinical practice, it is often by the pulsation on the apex of heart that TCM decides whether pectoral *qi* is weak or not.

3) Nourishing *Qi*

Nourishing *qi* refers to the *qi* circulating within the blood vessels and having a nourishing function.

As it flows through the vessels with blood, it has such a close relationship with the latter that TCM often mentions them in a combined way "nourishing blood". Compared with defending *qi*, nourishing *qi* belongs to *yin*, so it is also called "nourishing *yin*".

(1) Formation

Nourishing *qi* comes mainly from the food essence transformed and transported by the spleen and stomach. This is why a chapter on Arthralgia-Syndrome of ***Plain Questions*** says: "What is nourishing *qi* ? It is the essence of food and water."

(2) Movement

Nourishing *qi* originates from the middle warmer and enters the channels by way of the lung. It circulates throughout the body along one after another of the fourteen channels.

(3) Function

Nourishing *qi* has two main functions. One is to produce blood, that is, it flows into the channels through the lung and becomes a component of blood. The other is to nourish the whole body. That is, it goes up and down along the channels, circulating round the body and thus providing nutrients for the physiological activities of all the viscera and bowels, channels and collaterals, tissues and other organs. So, a chapter on the Pathogens Attacking the Body of ***Plain Questions*** says: "Nourishing *qi* secretes its fluid, which enters the channels and turns into blood, thus nourishing the limbs, the five viscera

中医常通过诊察“虚里”(相当于心尖搏动处)的搏动状况以测知宗气的盛衰。

3）营气

营气乃指运行脉中、具有营养作用的气。由于营气与血同行脉中，关系密切，故中医常“营血”并称。营气与卫气相对而言属于阴，故又称为“营阴”。

(1)生成

营气主要由脾胃运化的水谷精微所化生。故《素问·痹论》说：“营者，水谷之精气也。”

(2)运行

营气出于中焦，经肺进入经脉，沿十四经脉依次循行，周流全身。

(3)功能

营气的功能主要有二：一是化生血液，即营气经肺注入脉中，成为血液的组成部分；二是营养全身，即营气循脉上下，流注全身，为各脏腑、经络、组织、器官的生理活动提供营养。故《素问·邪客》说：“营气者，泌其津液，注之于脉，化以为血，以荣

and the six bowels."

4) Defending *Qi*

Defending *qi* is the *qi* moving outside the conduits and having protective functions. Compared with nourishing *qi*, it belongs to *yang*, so it is also known as "defending *yang*".

(1) Formation

Defending *qi* also comes from the food essence transformed and transported by the spleen and stomach. It is characterized by braveness in defence. That is why a chapter on Arthralgia-Syndrome of ***Plain Questions*** says: "Defending *qi* is a brave kind, which is produced by food and water."

(2) Movement

Defending *qi* circulates not within but outside the channels. Being vaporized to the diaphragm and scattered in the chest and abdomen, it travels between the skin and flesh. In spite of circualting outside the channels, it still leans against the channels when moving.

(3) Function

Defending *qi* has three functions. The first is guarding the surface of the body against exopathogen. The second is keeping a relatively constant body temperature by controlling the opening and closing of the pores and adjusting the excretion of sweat. The third is nourishing the viscera, bowels, muscles, skin and hair.

In addition, the circulation of defending *qi* is associated with sleep. Man goes to sleep when defending *qi* circulates in the interior of the body, whereas he wakes up when it circulates on the surface of the body.

When defending *qi* is insufficient, the defending function of the human body is weakened, the exopathogen invades the body easily, and the disease is hard to cure. Abnormal circulation of defending *qi* may cause sleep disorders. The longer defending *qi* circulates on the surface of the body, the shorter

四末，内注五脏六腑。”

4）卫气

卫气是运行于脉外，具有保卫功能的气。卫气与营气相对而言属于阳，故又称“卫阳”。

（1）生成

卫气亦由脾胃运化的水谷精气所化生，并具有“慓疾滑利”的特性，故《素问·痹论》说：“卫者，水谷之悍气也。”

（2）运行

卫气的循行，不受脉管的约束，行于脉外。在内则熏于肓膜，散于胸腹；在外则循皮肤之中，分肉之间。卫气虽行于脉外，但仍依傍着经脉而运行。

（3）功能

卫气的功能有三：一是护卫肌表，防御外邪入侵；二是调节、控制汗孔的开合、汗液的排泄，以维持体温的相对恒定；三是温养脏腑、肌肉、皮毛等。

此外，卫气循行与人的睡眠有关。当卫气行于体内时，人便入睡；行于体表，人便醒寝。

如卫气不足，人体防御功能低下，易被外邪侵袭，且病后难愈。若卫气循行异常，可出现寝寐异常。如卫气行于阳分（体表）

the duration of sleep, while the longer it circulates in the interior of the body, the longer the duration of sleep.

Nourishing *qi* and defending *qi* have the same source. The former circulates within the channels, has the nourishing function and belongs to *yin*, whereas the latter circulates outside the channels, has the function of guarding the exterior of the body and belongs to *yang*. Only when they coordinate with each other can the opening and closing of the pores be kept normal, the body temperature constant, and the defending ability strong. When they can not coordinate with each other because of an attack by exopathogen, such symptoms as aversion to wind, fever and sweating will occur.

Section 2
Blood

1. The Concept of Blood

Blood is a kind of red liquid rich in nutrition, circulating within the blood vessels. And vessels are pipes through which blood flows. So the book ***Plain Questions*** says in one of its chapters Essentials of Sphygmology: "Vessels serve as the reservoir of blood."

2. The Formation of Blood

Blood originates from two sources. One is food essence. The food essence developed in the spleen and stomach goes up to the lung where it is turned into blood through the efforts of the heart and lung. The other is the essence of life. This is proved by ***Plain Questions*** when it says in a chapter on Relevant Adaptation of the Human Body to Natural Environment: "The essence of life stored in the kidney goes into the bones and turns into marrow" and again says: "Strong marrows are sufficient to turn out vital energy and blood."

时间长则少寐，行于阴分时间长则多寐。

营气和卫气同出一源，但营行脉中，卫行脉外；营主营养而属阴，卫主卫外而属阳。二者相互协调，才能维持汗孔的正常开合、体温的恒定以及正常的防御能力。如为外邪所中，营卫不和，可出现恶风、发热、汗出等。

第二节　血

1. 血的概念

血是循行于脉管中富有营养作用的赤色液体。脉是血液循行的管道，故《素问·脉要精微论》说："夫脉者，血之府也。"

2. 血的生成

血液的生成主要有两种方式：一是水谷精微化血，即由脾胃化生的水谷精微上注于肺，通过心、肺的气化作用化生为血；二是精能化血，即《素问·生气通天论》所说"肾之精，并注于骨，而

This point is also illustrated by the book ***Zhang's Treatise on General Medicine***, written by Zhang Lu in 1695 A.D., when it says: "The stored essence of life goes into the liver and changes into clear blood."

As food essence developed in the spleen and stomach is the main source of blood, then the nutritional value of diet and the strength or weakness of the spleen and / or stomach will exert a direct influence on the formation of blood. This is why, in the treatment of patients whose blood is insufficient, TCM often administers some tonics which have the function of invigorating the spleen and stomach. For example, the book ***The Complete Effective Prescriptions for Women***, written by Chen Ziming in 1239 A.D. says: "Reinforcing the functions of the spleen and stomach causes blood to be developed spontaneously."

3. The Functions of Blood

Blood has the functions of nourishing and moistening the whole body. It circulates continuously, within the vessels, to the five viscera and six bowels in the interior, and to the skin, muscles, tendons and bones in the exterior, permanently providing nutrients for all the tissues and organs of the whole body so as to maintain their normal physiological functions. The book ***Plain Questions*** says in its chapter The Growth of the Five Viscera): "The liver having received blood has the function of determining good eyesight. The feet nourished by blood have the ability to walk. The palms having received blood have the power of gripping. The fingers having obtained nutrients from blood can hold objects." The book ***Miraculous Pivot*** says in the chapter The Internal Organs: "The normal blood makes the tendons and bones strong and the joints well lubricated." All these show that the sensation and movement of the body depend on the nutrients provided by blood.

Blood is the material basis for mental activity. Normal

为髓"，"骨髓坚固，气血随从"；《张氏医通》说："精不泄，归精于肝而化清血。"

由于脾胃化生的水谷精微是化生血液的主要资源，故饮食营养的优劣和脾胃功能的强弱，能直接影响血液的化生。中医在治疗血虚病人时常加用健脾和胃之品，其道理就在于此。如《妇人大全良方》说："补脾和胃，血自生矣。"

3．血的功能

血有营养、滋润全身的功能。血在脉中循行，内至五脏六腑，外达皮肉筋骨，如环无端，不断地为全身各组织、器官提供营养，以维持其正常的生理功能。《素问·五脏生成篇》说："肝受血而能视，足受血而能步，掌受血而能握，指受血而能摄。"《灵枢·本脏》说："血和则……筋骨劲强，关节清利矣"等，都说明机体的感觉和运动，必须由血提供营养才能进行。

血是神志活动的物质基础。血液供应充足，血脉运动正常，

mental activity depends on the normal circulation and a sufficient supply of blood. For example, The Formation and Movement of Nourishing and Defending *Qi*, a chapter of the book ***Miraculous Pivot*** syas: "The blood is the mental energy."

The Fast by Healthy Person, a chapter of the book ***Miraculous Pivot*** says: "Sufficient blood and healthy vessels lead to being full of vigour." So blood trouble caused by any kind of disorder may lead to signs and symptoms of mental illness, varying in degree. For example, deficiency of the blood of the heart may cause insomnia, dream-disturbed sleep and amnesia. The attack on the blood chamber by the exogenous pathogenic heat during menstruation may cause the patient to lapse into delirium in the evening as if she were seeing a ghost, while she may be lucid during the day.

4. The Circulation of Blood

The blood continuously circulates within the vessels round the body. As to how it circulates, there is an account in the book "***Plain Questions***, which states in a chapter On Channels: "The food is taken into the stomach; the food essence absorbed makes its way to the liver, ... then to the heart, nourishing the blood vessels, within which it (food essence) circulates to the lung; the blood flow of the whole body converges in the lung, from which it (food essence) is transported to the skin and hair, from where it (food essence) joints the essence of life in the blood capillaries and turns to the bowels and the four viscera". In spite of the fact that this original text deals mainly with the direction in which food essence circulates, it also sheds light on the direction of blood circulation.

The normal circulation of blood results from the mutual action of the heart, lung, spleen and liver. The heart controls the power to force blood to circulate. The lung is in charge of vital energy and linked to the formation of pectoral *qi*. The pectoral *qi* performs one of its functions when entering into the

神志活动才能正常。如《灵枢·营卫生会》说："血者，神气也。"《灵枢·平人绝谷》云："血脉和利，精神乃居。"故各种原因致成的血液异常，均可出现不同程度的神志症状。如心血虚，可见失眠、多梦、健忘等；热入血室，可出现昼日明了，暮则谵语，如见鬼状等。

4．血的循行

血液循行于脉管之中，流布全身，环周不休。关于血液循行的具体走向，在《素问·经脉别论》中有这样一段记载："食气入胃，散精于肝，……浊气归心，淫精于脉，脉气流经，经气归于肺，肺朝百脉，输精于皮毛，毛脉合精，行气于府，府精神明，留于四脏。"这段原文虽主要描述了水谷精气的运行方向，但可使我们从中了解血液循行的大体走向。

血液的正常循环，是心、肺、脾、肝共同作用的结果。心主血脉，心气是推动血液循行的基本动力；肺主气，与宗气生成有

heart channel to promote the movement of blood and vital energy. The spleen has the function of keeping the blood flowing within, not extravasating, the vessels. The liver has the functions of smoothing and regulating the flow of vital energy and blood, and storing the blood. It can regulate the rate of the flow of the blood within the vessels according to the different physiological needs of activity or calmness, causing the circulation of blood to be kept at a constant level. When the function of any one of the organs mentioned above is in disorder, the abnormal circulation of blood will occur. For example, a deficiency of the *qi* (vital energy) of the heart and lung may lead to the stagnation of the blood of the heart; a deficiency of the *qi* (vital energy) of the spleen impairs the spleen's function of keeping the blood flowing within the vessels, causes the blood to extravasate and leads to various kinds of hemorrhage. That the liver can't serve to regulate the activity of vital energy and blood may cause their stagnation.

Also, whether the vessels are free or not exerts a direct influence on the circulation of blood, as does a change in the temperature of blood.

Section 3
Jinye (Body Fluid)

1. The Concept of *Jinye* (Body Fluid)

What is "*jinye*" ? It is a collective term of all normal liquids. Its English equivalent is body fluid, which refers to the intracellular and the extracellular fluid in modern medicine.

Generally speaking, body fluid is subdivided into two kinds. "*Jin*" is the fluid which is dilute, flows easily in the pores, skin and muscles, and has a moistening function. "*Ye*" is the fluid which is thick, flows less easily in the joints, viscera, bowels,

关，而宗气的功能之一，就是贯心脉以行血气；脾统血，使血液循行于脉管之中而不外溢；肝主疏泄，有调畅气血运行的作用，并能藏血，可根据人体动与静的不同生理需要，调节脉管中的血流量，使血液循行保持恒定的水平。若以上某一脏器功能紊乱，均有可能导致血行异常。如心、肺气虚，运血无力，可致"心血瘀阻"；脾气虚弱，不能统血，可引起血液外溢而出现各种出血；肝失疏泄，气血运行不畅，可致气滞血瘀。

此外，脉管是否通利，血或寒或热，都能直接影响血液的运行。

第三节　津液

1．津液的概念

何谓津液？津液是人体内一切正常水液的总称。它包括现代医学所称的细胞内液和细胞外液。

一般来说，津液中性质较清稀，流动性较大，布散于皮肤、肌肉和孔窍等处，起滋润作用的，称为津；性质较稠厚，流动性

brain and marrow, and has a nourishing function. But in fact these two fluids are hard to separate completely and that is why they are combined into one expression "*jinye*".

2. The Formation, Distribution and Excretion of *Jinye* (Body Fluid)

"*Jinye*" comes from water and food. It is formed in the process of digestion in the stomach and transformation of the spleen. In addition, both the function of the small intestine in differentiating pure substance from turbid one and that of the large intestine in absorbing water from stool have something to do with the formation. So there exists the saying: "The small intestine has a function of, and the large intestine promotes, the formation of body fluid."

The transportation and distribution of body fluid is, in the main, completed jointly by the spleen through its function of transmission and transportation, by the lung through its efforts of dispersing and descending, and by the kidney through its role of regulating water metabolism. The triple warmer is the passage through which *jinye* passes. In addition, the liver's function of smoothing and regulating the flow of vital energy and blood also helps transport and distribute *jinye*. The heart plays a part in the transportation and distribution of *jinye*, for it controls the circulation of blood, of which *jinye* is a component. By way of the complex actions of viscera and bowels mentioned above, *jinye* can reach the skin, hair and muscles in the exterior, and the five viscera and six bowels in the interior, moisturizing all the tissues and organs round the body. This is what is called "*jinye* goes everywhere in the body by traveling along the channels of the five viscera."

The excretion of waste and excessive water in the body is often carried out according to different physiological needs. Some is sent, by the lung's function of activating the flow of body fluid, to the surface of the body and, is there turned into

较小，灌注于骨节、脏腑、脑、髓等处，起濡养作用的，称为液。实际上津与液很难截然分开，故多津液并称。

2．津液的生成、输布与排泄

津液来源于饮食水谷，通过胃的“游溢”、脾的“散精”而生成。此外，小肠的“分清别浊”、大肠的吸收水液功能，也与津液生成有关，故有“小肠主液”、“大肠主津”之说。

津液的输布，主要靠脾的转输、肺的宣降和肾的气化作用来完成。三焦是水液通行的道路。此外，肝的疏泄作用亦有助于津液的输布。津液是血液的主要成分，心主行血，亦与津液输布有关。通过以上脏腑的综合作用，津液可外达肌腠皮毛，内注五脏六腑，滋润全身各组织、器官。此即所谓“水精四布，五经并行”。

体内无用、多余水液的排泄，常根据机体的不同生理需要，

sweat. Some is changed into urine by the kidney's function of separating the clear from the turbid and removed by the urinary bladder's function of storing and excreting urine. Others are transformed into nasal mucus, saliva and tears and are removed from the nose, mouth, eyes by the functions of the corresponding organs. Also, the air exhaled by the lung takes away some moisture.

In short, the formation, distribution and excretion of "*jinye*" is a complicated process which needs the coordinated work of many organs. Therefore, the pathological changes in many viscera and bowels may all affect the normal metabolism of "*jinye*". For instance, an excessive loss of "*jinye*" will result in its perishing. Disturbances in the transportation, distribution and excretion of "*jinye*" may cause the stagnation of water, which is manifested by phlegm-retention diseases and edema. Pathological changes of "*jinye*" will also affect the functions of many viscera and bowels. For example, damage of "*jinye*" and dryness of the lung cause dry cough; heart trouble caused by the retention of water is marked by palpitation; the pathological accumulation of fluid in the lung leads to dyspnea or cough. In the treatment of the above disorders, TCM always pays much attention to recuperating the lung, the spleen and the kidney, for it believes that they are key organs in maintaining the normal metabolism of water.

3. The Functions of Body Fluid

1) Moisturizing and Nourishing

The "*jinye*" distributed to the surface and pores of the body has the function of moisturizing the skin, the hair, the muscles, the eyes, the nose, the mouth and others. "*Jinye*" poured into the internal organs, the marrow, the spinal cord and the brain has the function of nourishing them.

有的通过肺的宣发作用输送至体表化为汗；有的则通过肾和膀胱的气化作用化为尿；还有的通过相关脏器的作用转为涕、唾、泪，从鼻、口、目排出体外。此外，肺在呼气中亦能带走部分水分。

总之，津液的生成、输布与排泄是一个复杂的过程，需要许多脏腑的参与与协调才能完成。因此，许多脏腑的病变都可影响津液的正常代谢。如津液丧失过多，就会亡津；输布、排泄障碍，就会水液停滞，出现痰饮、水肿。津液的病变也会影响许多脏腑的功能，如津伤肺燥则干咳，水气凌心则心悸，饮邪射肺则喘咳。由于中医认为肺、脾、胃三脏是维持津液正常代谢的关键，故在治疗时多以调理肺、脾、肾为主。

3．津液的功能

1）滋润、濡养

被输布于体表、孔窍等处的津，能滋润皮毛、肌肤、目、鼻、口等；被灌注于内脏、骨髓、脊髓、脑等处的液，能濡养内脏，充养骨髓、脊髓和脑等。

2) As a Component of Blood

"*Jinye*" seeps into the blood vessels through the blood capillaries, performs a nourishing and lubricating function and becomes a component part of blood.

As is known, the physiological needs in the body and the climatic changes in the external world are often followed by corresponding physiological changes in the metabolism of body fluid. For example, if you wear more clothes on a hot day, you will sweat, giving off the heat in your body. If you wear less clothes on a cold day, you will not sweat, and that part of liquid will turn into urine that is yet to be discharged. This helps maintain your body temperature.

When *jinye* metabolizes, it can also cause the waste formed after metabolism in the body, and poisonous substances to leave the body along with sweat and urine, thus maintaining the clearness of the body itself and ensuring the normal physiological functions of the viscera, bowels, channels and collaterals, tissues and other organs.

Section 4
The Relationship between *Qi* Blood and Body Fluid

Qi, blood and body fluid have different properties, forms and functions but have something in common. To begin with, they are the basic materials that comprise the human body and keep the body's life activities ongoing. Secondly, they all derive from food essence. Thirdly, they physiologically depend on each other for their existence and they restrain and utilize each other. And lastly, they influence each other and have causality between each other in the pathological field. There-

2）化生血液

津液经孙络渗入血脉之中，具有滋养、滑利血脉的作用，并成为血液的主要组成部分。

此外，津液的代谢常随体内生理需要和外界气候变化而发生相应的生理变化，如天暑衣厚，则汗出，以散热；天寒衣薄，则汗止，而化为尿，以保存体温。这有助于保持体温的恒定。

津液在其自身的代谢过程中，还能把机体的代谢废物及有毒物质随汗、尿等排出体外，以保持人体本身的自洁，使脏腑、经络、组织、器官始终保持正常的生理功能。

第四节　气、血、津液的关系

气、血、津液的性状及其功能虽各有其特点，但三者均是构成人体和维持人体生命活动的最基本物质。它们在生成方面，均离不开水谷精气；在生理方面，相互依存，相互制约和相互为用；在病理方面，亦互相影响，互为因果。因而在治疗时，就应

fore, when treating diseases related to them, the relationship between them must be considered.

1. The Relationship between *Qi* and Blood

Qi belongs to *yang* and has a warming function; while blood belongs to *yin*, and has a nourishing function. These are the differences between the two in property and function. What is more, there is such a close relationship between *qi* and blood that "the *qi* is 'the commander' of blood " and "blood is 'the mother' of *qi*.", which can be explained as follows:

1) *Qi* as the Commander of Blood

The meaning of *qi* as the commander of blood contains the following three aspects:

(1) Making Blood

Qi is the motive power for making blood. *Qi* is indispensable when water and food are changed into food essence; food essence is then changed into nourishing *qi* and body fluid; nourishing *qi* and body fluid are turned into red blood; the essence of life is changed into blood, and marrow transforms into blood. The functions of *qi* mentioned above, however, are performed mainly by the functional activities of the relevant viscera and bowels. When *qi* is sufficient, the functional activities of the viscera and bowels are full of vigour, and the ability to make blood is also strong. When *qi* is insufficient, the functional activities of the viscera and bowels are weak, and the ability to make blood is also weak. Therefore, a deficiency of *qi* often leads to a more deficiency of blood. The deficiency of both *qi* and blood gives rise to such symptoms and signs as shortness of breath, lassitude, pale complexion, dizziness, dim eyesight, palpitation and others. In treating a deficiency of blood, TCM often adds drugs having the function of invigorating *qi* to those having the function of enriching blood. For example, Chinese Angelica Decoction for Replenishing Blood is one of

充分考虑它们的相互关系。

1．气与血的关系

气属阳，主煦之；血属阴，主濡之。这是二者在属性、功能上的差别。但气血之间，又存在着“气为血之帅”、“血为气之母”的密切关系。现分述如下：

1）气为血之帅

气为血之帅有以下三方面的含义：

（1）气能生血

是说气是血液生成的动力。从摄入饮食物到转化成水谷精微；从水谷精微转化为营气、津液；从营气、津液转化为赤色血液，以及精髓化血等，无不依赖气的作用。而气的这些作用，主要是通过有关脏腑的功能活动来实现的。气足，则脏腑的功能活动旺盛，化生血液的能力亦强；气虚，则脏腑功能活动减弱，化生血液的能力亦弱。所以，气虚常可进一步导致血虚，而见气短、乏力、面色苍白、头晕、眼花、心悸等气血两虚的病症。中医在

the prescriptions which functions well in enriching blood. It consists of 6 grams of Chinese angelica root (*Radix Angelicae Sinensis*) which has the property of enriching blood, and 30 grams of milkvetch root (*Radix Astragali seu Hedysari*) which has the function to invigorate *qi*. Why ? Because *qi* has the function of promoting the development of blood.

(2) *Qi* as the Driving Force of Blood

Qi is also the motivating power which propels blood forward. On the one hand, it can propel blood forward directly, which is, what is called, "*qi* in motion renders blood circulating normally." On the other hand, it can drive blood forward indirectly by means of the functions of the relevant viscera and bowels, such as driving function of the *qi* of the heart, dispersing function of the *qi* of the lung, and smoothing and regulating functions of the *qi* of the liver. Therefore, the stagnation or deficiency of *qi*, or the disorder of the relevant viscera and bowels, can block the flow of blood, and even cause blood stasis. So when treating the syndromes that are due to blood stasis, TCM not only prescribes drugs having the property of promoting blood circulation and resolving blood stasis, but also adds drugs having the property of promoting the circulation of, or supplementing *qi*, according to different causes. Meanwhile, it pays attention to recuperating the functions of the relevant viscera and bowels.

(3) Keeping Blood Flowing within the Vessels

Qi (vital energy) has the function of keeping blood circulating normally within, not extravasating, the vessels. This function of *qi* is mainly based on the function of the spleen. For example, when *qi* is insufficient, especially when the spleen fails to keep blood flowing within the vessels, various kinds of hemorrhage often occur. When treating them, TCM is not for using excessive hemostatics but mainly for using drugs having the function of invigorating the spleen to benefit *qi* such as ginseng root (*Radix Ginseng*), milkvetch root (*Radix Astragali*

治疗血虚时，常于补血药中，配以补气之品。如当归补血汤，该方由具有补血作用的当归6克和具有补气作用的黄芪30克组成，即取“气能生血”之意。

(2)气能行血

气也是推动血液循行的动力。气一方面能直接推动血行，即所谓“气行则血行”；另一方面，又可通过有关脏腑的功能来推动血行，如心气的推动、肺气的敷布、肝气的疏泄等。因此，不论是气滞、气虚，还是相关脏腑功能失调，都可引起血行不利，甚至导致血瘀。故中医在治疗瘀血证时，不仅使用活血化瘀药，而且还根据其具体原因，分别加用行气或益气之品，并注意调理有关脏腑的功能。

(3)气能摄血

气有统摄血液，使之在脉管中正常循行而不外溢的作用。气的这一作用，主要通过脾气的功能来实现。如气虚，特别是脾气虚不能统血，常导致各种出血证。中医治疗时并不主张用过多的

seu Hedysari), large-headed atractylodes rhizome (*Rhizoma Atractylodis Macrocephalae*) and licorice root (*Radix Glycyrrhizae*). In so doing, the hemostatic aim may be attained by recuperating the spleen's function of keeping blood flowing within the vessels.

2) Blood as "the Mother" of *Qi*

The concept of blood as "the mother" of *qi* has two aspects. One is that *qi* is in blood and carried by blood. The other is that blood permanently provides nutrients for the movement of *qi*. Therefore, *qi* can not exist without blood. That is why those whose blood is deficient have deficient *qi*. Those who have lost a lot of blood have less *qi*. Because of this, in the treatment, *qi* should be reinforced at the same time as blood is toned up, and vice versa.

2. The Relationship between *Qi* and Body Fluid

The relationship between *qi* and body fluid is quite similar to that between *qi* and blood, and may be summarized into the following four aspects.

1) *Qi*, the Motivating Power in Promoting the Development of Body Fluid

Qi is also the motivating power in the development of body fluid. Body fluid is developed mainly through the functions of the spleen and stomach. It, however, has the ability to promote the functions of the spleen and stomach. So, when *qi* is sufficient, the functions of the spleen and stomach are sound, and the body fluid is abundant. When *qi* is deficient, the functions of the spleen and stomach are weakened, and the body fluid is insufficient.

止血药，而且主要选用人参、黄芪、白术、甘草等补脾益气药，通过恢复脾统血的功能来达到止血之目的。

2）血为气之母

血为气之母有两个含义：一是气存血中，血以载气；二是血始终为气的运动提供营养物质。所以，气不能离开血液而单独存在。故血虚者，气亦虚；血脱者，气亦脱。治疗亦互相兼顾，其道理即在于此。

2．气与津液的关系

气与津液的关系和气与血的关系极其雷同，可归纳为以下四个方面：

1）气能生津

气也是津液化生的动力。津液主要通过脾胃的功能而生成，而气有推动脾胃功能的作用。所以，气旺，则脾胃功能健旺，化生的津液就充盛；气虚，则脾胃功能减弱，化生的津液就不足。

2) *Qi*, the Motivating Power in Promoting the Circulation of Body Fluid and the Excretion of Water

The ascending, descending, exiting and entering of *qi* is the motivating power for body fluid to be transported, distributed and excreted, There is a saying: "*Qi* has the function of promoting the circulation of body fluid and the excretion of water." Of course, *Qi* performs this function with the help of the lung, spleen, kidney, triple warmer, urinary bladder and relevant viscera or bowels. Therefore, a deficiency or stagnation of *qi* or abnormal functions of the relevant viscera or bowels caused by any factor may lead to a disturbance in transporting, distributing and excreting body fluid, which is known as "*qi* fails to promote the circulation of body fluid" and "*qi* is unable to help excrete water." Promoting the circulation of or supplementing *qi* and promoting diuresis are good measures to be taken in solving this problem. Meanwhile, the functions of the relevant viscera or bowels should be restored.

3) *Qi*, the Mechanism of Guiding Body Fluid

The guiding action of *qi* can regulate and control the excretion of body fluid. The balance of the metabolism of fluid in the body can be kept only by this action of *qi*. If *qi* fails to control the excretion of body fluid, the body fluid will flow away without reason. For example, if defending *qi* cannot function well in regulating body fluid, spontaneous sweating will occur; if the kidney's *qi* is insufficient in controlling body fluid, there will occur enuresis and polyuria. In the clinical treatment of these disorders, the method of invigorating *qi* to control body fluid is often used.

4) Body Fluid, The Carrier of *Qi*

Body fluid is also the carrier of *qi*. *Qi* exists through its

2）气能行津、化水

气的升降出入是津液输布、排泄的动力。故有“气能行津”、“气能化水”的说法。当然，气的行津、化水功能，主要是通过肺、脾、肾、三焦、膀胱等有关脏腑的气化功能来实现。因此，当某种原因造成气虚、气滞或相关脏腑气化功能失调时，均可导致津液的输布、排泄障碍，称作“气不行津”、“气不化水”，治疗时多行气或益气与利水法并用，并同时调理有关脏腑的气化功能。

3）气能摄津

气的固摄作用能调节、控制津液的排泄。体内的津液只有在气的这一作用下才能维持其代谢平衡。若气的固摄作用减弱，就会导致体内津液无故流失。如卫气不固则自汗，肾气不足则遗尿、多尿等。临床治疗多用补气固津法。

4）津能载气

津液亦是气的载体，气依附于津液而存在。因此，津液的流

attachment to body fluid. Therefore, the loss of body fluid often damages *qi*. For example, over-sweating or profuse sweating may damage *qi*. Repeated severe vomiting and diarrhea cause heavy loss of body fluid, which, in turn, give rise to heavy loss of *qi*. This is the reason why You Zaijing, a medical man in the Qing dynasty, says in his book ***The Essence of the Synopsis of the Golden Chamber***: "After vomiting, no one has perfect *qi*."

3. The Relationship between Blood and Body Fluid

Blood and body fluid are both liquid substances. Their main function is nourishing and moisturizing. And they both belong to *yin*.

Both blood and body fluid derive from food essence. Fluid in the body seeps constantly into the blood vessels and becomes a component of blood. Blood extravasates out of the blood vessels and turns into body fluid. And this is the resaon why there is such a saying: "Body fluid and blood have the same source."

So pathologically, whenever there is not enough blood, body fluid, in turn, becomes less. In this case, dry skin, even dry nails will occur. Heavy losses of blood are followed by heavy losses of body fluid. This will cause thirst, oliguria and dry skin. Less body fluid causes blood to be less but thicker. As sweat comes from body fluid, and "blood and sweat have the same source", the book "*Ling Shu*" (***Miraculous Pivot***) says in the chapter Formation and Movement of Nourishing *Qi* and Defending *Qi*: "Those who suffer from blood loss hardly perspire. Those who perspire a lot have less blood than normal." The book ***Treatise on Febrile Diseases*** also warns, "Those who are afflicted with hemorrhage should free themselves from perspiring. Those whose blood loss is too heavy have to avoid perspiring."

失亦常带来气的损伤。如发汗太过、大汗淋漓，可导致气的损伤；频繁、大量的呕吐、腹泻，不仅丧失津液，亦可出现“气随津脱”。故清·尤在泾在《金匮要略心典》中说：“吐下之余，定无完气。”

3．血与津液的关系

血与津液，均为液态物质，都以营养、滋润为其主要功用。与气相对而言，皆属于阴。

血与津液同源于水谷精微。分布于全身各组织中的津液不断地渗入孙络，即成为血液的组成部分；而运行于络脉中的血液如渗出脉外，便成为津液，故有“津血同源”之说。

因此，在病理上，血液不足，津液亦乏，可见肌肤干燥，甚至甲错；失血过多，津液亦亡，必见口渴、尿少、皮肤干燥；津液外亡，亦会使血液枯稠。由于汗为津液所化，“血汗同源”，故《灵枢·营卫生会》说：“夺血者无汗，夺汗者无血。”《伤寒论》中亦有“衄家不可发汗”、“亡血家不可发汗”之诫。

Chapter Five
The Theory of the Channels and Collaterals

The theory of channels and collaterals concerns the study of the physiology and pathology of the channels and collaterals, and their mutual relations. It is as essential a part of the basic theory of TCM as the theory of *yin* and *yang*, five elements, viscera, *qi*, blood and body fluid.

It forms the basis of all clinical departments of TCM, especially of acupuncture, moxibustion and massage. Anyone who wants to have a good command of the above skills must have a good grasp of this theory first.

Section 1
The Concept and Content of the Channels and Collaterals

1. The Concept of the Channels and Collaterals

What is meant by the channel and collateral ? The channel, or "*jing*" in Chinese, means route, and is the main trunk running lengthways in the system of the channels and collaterals; while the collateral, or "*luo*" in Chinese, means net, and is the branch of a channel in the system.

TCM holds that the channels and collaterals are distributed over the whole body. They are linked with each other and connect the superficial, interior, upper and lower portions of the human body, making the body an organic whole.

第五章

经络学说

经络学说是研究经络的生理、病理及其相互关系的学说。同阴阳、五行、脏腑、气血津液学说一样，它也是中医基本理论的重要组成部分。

经络学说是中医临床各科，特别是针灸、推拿的理论基础。凡欲精此术者，必须首先弄通这一学说。

第一节　经络的概念与组成

1．经络的概念

何谓经络？经，在汉语里有路径之意，它是经络系统纵行的主干；络，在汉语里有网络之意，它是经络系统的分支。

中医认为，人体经络遍及全身，相互贯通，从而把人体的内、外、上、下，联结成了一个有机的整体。

2. The Composition of the Channels and Collaterals

The system of the channels and collaterals consists of channels, collaterals and their subsidiary parts.

The channels may be divided into regular channels and extra channels. There are twelve regular channels, including three *yin* channels of the hand and foot, and three *yang* channels of the hand and foot. They are referred to altogether as the Twelve Channels. The Eight Extra Channels consist of what is called the *Du* Channel, the *Ren* Channel, the *Chong* Channel, the *Dai* Channel, the *Yinqiao* Channel, the *Yangqiao* Channel, the *Yinwei* Channel and *Yangwei* Channel. They are commonly referred to as the Eight Extra Channels.

The collaterals can be classified as the reticular branch conduits, superficial collaterals, and small collaterals. All the Twelve Channels, and the *Du* and the *Ren* Channels have one reticular branch conduit each. These reticular branch conduits and the great reticular conduit of the spleen add up to fifteen. The superficial collaterals are the ones that run in the surface layer of the human body, and often make their appearance on the surface. The small collaterals are the finest.

In addition, there are internal branches, tendons and skin zone of the Twelve Channels in the system of the channels and collaterals. Following is a more detailed description given of the Twelve Channels and the Eight Extra Channels because of their important place.

2. 经络的组成

经络系统是由经脉、络脉及其连属部分组成的。

经可分为正经、奇经二类。正经有十二，包括手、足三阴经和手、足三阳经，合称十二经脉。奇经有八，即由督脉、任脉、冲脉、带脉、阴跷脉、阳跷脉、阴维脉、阳维脉组成，合称奇经八脉。

络有别络、浮络、孙络之分。十二经脉和督、任二脉各有一支别络，再加上脾之大络，合为十五别络。浮络是循行于人体浅表部位而常浮现的络脉。孙络则是最细小的络脉。

此外，在经络系统中，还有十二经别、十二经筋和十二皮部。由于十二经脉、奇经八脉在经络系统中最为常用，故仅将其介绍如下：

Section 2
The Twelve Channels

1. The Classification and Name of the Twelve Channels

Classification of the Twelve Channels

Three *Yin* Channels of Hand	The Lung Channel of Hand-*Taiyin* The Pericardium Channel of Hand-*Jueyin* The Heart Channel of Hand-*Shaoyin*
Three *Yang Channels* of Hand	The Large Intestine Channel of Hand-*Yangming* The Triple Warmer Channel of Hand-*Shaoyang* The Small Intestine Channel of Hand *Taiyang*
Three *Yin* Channels of Foot	The Spleen Channel of Foot-*Taiyin* The Liver Channel of Foot-*Jueyin* The Kidney Channel of Foot-*Shaoyin*
Three *Yang* Channels of Foot	The Stomach Channel of Foot-*Yangming* The Gall Bladder Channel of Foot-*Shaoyang* The Urinary Bladder Channel of Foot-*Taiyang*

The above list shows that the full name of a channel is composed of the following three parts:

1) Hand or Foot: The channels starting from or terminating at the hand are named "Hand", while those starting from or terminating at the foot are termed "Foot".

2) *Yin* or *Yang* : The channels running in the medial aspect of the extremities are called "*Yin*", whereas those in the lateral aspect are termed "*Yang*".

The medial aspect of the extremities can be subdivided into the anterior border,the mid-line and the posterior border, so the *yin* channels running through these parts are called *Tai-*

第二节　十二经脉

1. 十二经脉的分类与命名

十二经脉的分类

手三阴经	手太阴肺经 手厥阴心包经 手少阴心经
手三阳经	手阳明大肠经 手少阳三焦经 手太阳小肠经
足三阴经	足太阴脾经 足厥阴肝经 足少阴肾经
足三阳经	足阳明胃经 足少阳胆经 足太阳膀胱经

上表说明，每一经脉的全称，是由以下三部分组成：

1）手或足：起于或止于手的经脉，称之为“手”；而起于或止于足的经脉，则称之为“足”。

2）阴或阳：循行于肢体内侧面的经脉，称之为“阴”；而循行于肢体外侧面的则称之为“阳”。

由于肢体的内侧面又可再划分为前缘、中线和后缘，循行于这些部位的阴经则依次称之为“太阴”、“厥阴”和“少阴”；肢体的

yin, *Jueyin* and *Shaoyin* accordingly. The lateral aspect of the extremities can also be subdivided into the anterior border, the mid-line and the posterior border, so *yang* channels are termed "*Yangming*", "*Shaoyang*" and "*Taiyang*".

3) The Visceral Name: The visceral name of each channel is determined by the organ to which it pertains. For example, the channel pertaining to the lung is named the Lung Channel.

2. The Courses of the Twelve Channels and Their Pathological Symptoms

The descriptions concerning the courses of the Twelve Channels and their pathological symptoms in this book are mainly selected from the relevant text of On Channels, a chapter of ***Miraculous Pivot***, also known as ***Canon of Acupuncture*** (722–221 B.C.), which contains the earliest records on the courses of the Twelve Channels and their pathological symptoms. Of course, some necessary revisions have been made in terms of content.

1) The Lung Channel of Hand-*Taiyin*

(1) Course

The Lung Channel of Hand-*Taiyin* originates in the middle warmer, the portion between the diaphragm and the umbilicus of the body cavity, running downwards to communicate with the large intestine①. Turning back, it goes along the orifices of the stomach (the pylorus and cardia)②, then upwards through the diaphragm ③ into its pertaining organ, the lung④. From the pulmonary series (including the trachea, throat, etc.), it comes transversely to the armpit (out of Point Zhongfu, L1)⑤. It then descends along the medial aspect of the upper arm, and passes in front of the Heart Channel of Hand-*Shaoyin* and the Pericardium Channel of Hand-*Jueyin*⑥, down to the middle portion of the elbow⑦. From there it runs along the anterior

外侧面亦有前缘、中线和后缘之分，其名称则依次称之为“阳明”、“少阳”和“太阳”。

3）脏腑的名称：每一经脉的脏腑名称是依据该经所属的脏腑而定。例如，属于肺的经脉，就称之为“肺经”。

2．十二经脉的循行与病症

本书有关十二经脉的循行与病症的描述，主要选自《灵枢·经脉》(公元前722～221年)有关原文。此乃十二经脉循行及其病症的最早记载。当然，对其中的某些文字，亦做了必要的调整。

1）手太阴肺经

（1）循行

肺手太阴之脉，起于中焦，下络大肠①，还循胃口（幽门和贲门）②，上膈③，属肺④。从肺系(包括气管、咽喉等)，横出腋下(出自中府穴)⑤下循臑内(上臂内侧)，行少阴、心主（手少阴心经、手厥阴心包经)之前⑥，下肘中⑦，循臂内上骨下廉(前臂

border of the radius on the medial aspect of the forearm⑧ and goes into *Cunkou*, the place on the wrist over the radial artery where the pulse is felt⑨. Then it arrives at the thenar⑩, runs along its border⑪ and emerges from the medial side of the tip of the thumb (Point Shaoshang, Lu 11)⑫.

The branch of the channel runs directly from the proximal aspect of the wrist (Point Lieque, Lu 7) into the radial side of the tip of the index (Point Shangyang LI1), in which it connects with the Large Intestine Channel of Hand-*Yangming* (See Fig.1).

Note: The ordinal numbers in the circle on the foregoing paragraphs, i.e.,①, ②, ③, ... are in keeping with those marked in the figure attached to the end of the book. The same is true of the figures below.

(2) Pathological Symptoms

The primary symptom resulting from a disorder of the channel itself is lung-distension, characterized by dyspnea, cough, and pain in the supraclavicular fossa. The pain may be so sharp that the patient clasps his hands across the chest with blurred vision, which is named "*Bijue*" in TCM. A disorder of the channel, affected by lung disease, is symptomatized by cough, asthma, thirst, impatience, fullness in the chest, pain and a cold feeling along the anterior border of the medial aspect of the arm, and a burning sensation in the palms. One whose *qi* of the channel is excessive has a pain in the shoulder and the back, or coryza caused by wind and cold, or sweat due to catching pathogenic wind, or frequency of micturition and oliguria. One whose *qi* of the channel is deficient has a pain and cold feeling in the shoulder and the back, or has difficulty in breathing or the colour of his urine changes.

2) The Large Intestine Channel of Hand-*Yangming*

(1) Course

This channel starts from the tip of the radial side of the index (Point Shangyang, LI1)①. It runs upwards along the

内侧，桡骨前缘）⑧，入寸口⑨，上鱼⑩，循鱼际⑪，出大指之端（拇指内侧端，即少商穴）⑫。

其支者，从腕后（列缺穴）⑬直出次指内廉，出其端（食指桡侧端，即商阳穴），交手阳明大肠经（见图1）。

注：上文中序码，即①、②、③……，与本书末附图中的序号一致，下同。

（2）病症

是动（本经异常所发生的病症）则肺胀满，膨膨而喘咳，缺盆中痛，甚则交两手而瞀（两手抱胸而视物不清），此为"臂厥"。是主肺所生病者（因肺病影响而致该经异常所发生的病症），咳上气，喘，渴，烦心，胸满，臑臂内前廉痛厥，掌中热。气盛有余，则肩背痛，风寒，汗出中风，小便数而欠（小便频数而量少）；气虚则肩背痛寒，少气不足以息，溺色变。

2）手阳明大肠经

（1）循行

大肠手阳明之脉，起于大指次指之端（食指桡侧末端，即商

radial side of the index and passes between the ossa metacarpalia I and II, goes into the depression between the tendons of m. extensor pollicis longus and brevis, then along the antero-lateral aspect of the forearm[3] to the lateral side of the elbow (Point Quchi, LI11)[4]. Along the anterior border of the lateral side of the upper arm[5], it ascends to the highest point of the shoulder (Point Jianyu, LI15)[6], and then goes along the anterior border of the acromion[7] up to 7th cervical vertebra (Point Dazhui, Du 14)[8], from where it comes downwards into the supraclavicular fossa[9] and communicates with the lung[10]. Descending through the diaphragm[11], it enters its pertaining organ, the large intestine[12].

The branch channel from the supraclavicular fossa runs upwards to the neck[13], passes through the cheek[14], and enters into the lower teeth and gum[15]. Then it curves round the lips and meets at Point Renzhong (Du 26), or philtrum, the vertical groove on the mid-line of the upper lip. From there the channel of the left side turns right, while the right side channel turns left. They go upwards to both sides of the wings of the nose (Point Yingxiang LI20)[16] and connect with the Stomach Channel of Foot-*Yangming* (See Fig. 2).

(2) Pathological Symptoms

A disorder of the channel itself causes toothache and swelling of the neck. A disorder of the channel, which is caused by the disease of the large intestine and the pathometabolism of the body fluid the disease affects, gives rise to icteric sclera, dry mouth, epistaxis, pharyngitis, pain along the anterior border of the shoulder and the upper arm, and akinesia of the index finger. Those whose *qi* of the channel is excessive probably suffer from heat and swelling of the regions where the channel passed, while those whose *qi* of the channel is deficient often suffer from severe shivering.

3) The Stomach Channel of Foot-*Yangming*

(1) Course

阳穴)[1]，循指上廉(食指桡侧)，出合谷两骨之间(第一、二掌骨之间)，上入两筋之中（拇长伸肌腱与拇短伸肌腱之间)[2]，循臂上廉(前臂外侧前缘)[3]，入肘外廉(肘部外侧，即曲池穴处)[4]，上臑外前廉(上臂外侧前缘)[5]，上肩(肩髃穴)[6]，出髃骨之前廉(肩峰前缘)[7]，上出于柱骨之会上(大椎穴)[8]，下入缺盆（锁骨上窝)[9]，络肺[10]，下膈[11]，属大肠[12]。

其支者，从缺盆上颈[13]，贯颊[14]，入下齿中[15]，还出挟口，交人中，左之右(左脉向右)，右之左(右脉向左)，上挟鼻孔（分布在鼻翼两旁，即迎香)[16]，交足阳明胃经(见图2)。

(2)病症

是动则齿痛，颈肿。是主津液所生病者（大肠病及津液，进而影响经脉)，目黄，口干，鼽衄(鼻出血)，喉痹，肩前臑痛，大指次指(即食指)不用。气有余，则当脉所过者热肿，虚则寒栗不复。

3)足阳明胃经

(1)循行

This channel starts from the side of the nose (Point Yingxiang LI20), and ascends to the root of the nose[1], meeting the Urinary Bladder Channel (at Point Jingming, UB1)[2]. Then it descends along the lateral side of the nose[3] and enters into the upper gum[4]. Emerging and curving round the lips[5], it passes downwards and connects with the symmetrical channel at Point Chengjiang (Ren 24)[6] in the sulcus mentolabiabialis. And it runs along the posterior-inferior side of the parotid gland, through Point Daying (St 5)[7], and Point Jiache in (St 6) succession, and then ascends in front of the ear, through Point Kezhuren, i. e., Shangguan (GB 3), the point of the Gall Bladder Channel of Foot-*Shaoyang*[9]. And finally, it runs along the hairline[10] and reaches the forehead (Point Touwei, St 8)[11]

One of its branches sprouts in front of Daying (St 5), descends to Renying (St 9), and goes along the throat[12] into the supraclavicular fossa[13]. From there it descends through the diaphragm[14], enters into its pertaining organ, the stomach, and communicates with the spleen[15].

A straight branch from the supraclavicular fossa descends to the medial border of the papilla mammae[16]. Then it makes its descent along the side of the umbilicus and enters into Point Qijie i. e., Qichong (St 30)[17].

One of the branches starting from the pylorus descends through the abdominal cavity, and joins the straight branch at Point Qijie (St 30)[18]. From there it descends through Point Biguan (St 31)[19], Futu (St 35)[20], to the knee[21]. Along the anterolateral aspect of the tibia[22], it goes towards the dorsum of the foot[23], and then to the lateral side of the tip of the second toe (Point Lidui St 45)[24].

Another branch sprouting from the region 3 individual *cun* below the genu (Point Zusanli, St 36)[25], descends to the lateral side of the middle toe[26].

The branch sprouting from the dorsum of the foot (Point Chongyang, St 42) descends into the medial margin of the hal-

胃足阳明之脉，起于鼻之交頞中(鼻翼两侧，使迎香穴，上行至鼻根部)[1]，旁纳太阳之脉[2]，下循鼻外[3]，入上齿中[4]，还出挟口环唇[5]，下交承浆[6]，却循颐后下方(腮后下方)，出大迎[7]，循颊车[8]，上耳前，过客主人(即上关，为足少阳胆经穴)[9]，循发际[10]，至额颅(头维穴)[11]

其直者，从大迎前下人迎，循喉咙[12]，入缺盆[13]，下膈[14]，属胃，络脾[15]。

其支者，从缺盆下乳内廉[16]，下挟脐，入气街中(即气冲穴)[17]。

其支者，起于胃口，下循腹里，下至气街而合[18]。以下髀关[19]，抵伏兔[20]，下膝膑中[21]，下循胫外廉[22]，下足(足背)[23]，入中指内间(应作次趾外间，即足第二趾外侧端厉兑穴)[24]。

其支者，下廉三寸而别(足三里穴)[25]，下入中趾外间[26]。

其支者，别跗上(冲阳穴)，入大趾间，出其端(隐白穴)[27]，

lux, and through its tip (Point Yinbai, Sp 1)㉑, connects with the Spleen Channel of Foot *Taiyin* (See Fig. 3).

(2) Pathological Symptoms

A disorder of the channel itself causes the following symptoms: shivering with a feeling of cold water being sprinkled over the body, frequent groans, repeated yawns, and black and dark colour of the frontal skin. When a disease of the channel occurs, the patient is very much inclined to avoid meeting with people and fire. He is very likely to be startled on hearing a woody sound and prefers a solitary life. His condition may be so serious that he climbs to a height to sing aloud and runs about stark-naked. He has borborygmus and abdominal distension, which is called "*Ganjue*" in TCM. Some symptoms that may be present due to blood trouble caused by a disorder of the stomach are: mania, malaria, febrile disease, hidrosis, epistaxis, deviation of the mouth, lip boil, swelling of the neck, sorethroat, ascites, swelling and pain of the patella, pain along the course of the channel in the chest, breast, Qijie (St 30), thigh, Futu (St 32), the anterior-lateral aspect of the tibia and the dosum of the foot, and the akinesia of the middle toe. A patient whose *qi* of the channel is excessive may feel the heat in the anterior part of the body. Hyperfunction of the stomach will lead to rapid digestion, hunger, and yellowish urine. The patient whose *qi* of the channel is deficient may have frequent shiver in the anterior part of the body. If his stomach trouble is caused by pathogenic cold, he will have abdominal distension.

4) The Spleen Channel of Foot-*Taiyin*

(1) Course

The channel starts from the tip of the medial side of the great toe (Yinbai, Sp 1)①. From there it runs along the junction of the red and white skin of the medial aspect of the great toe, passes the posterior surface of "*Hegu*", the nodular process on the medial aspect of the first metatarsophalangeal joint②

交足太阴脾经(见图3)。

(2)病症

是动则病洒洒振寒，善伸(时常呻吟)，数欠(反复地打呵欠)，颜黑。病至则恶人与火，闻木声则惕然而惊，心欲动，独闭户塞牖而处，甚则欲上高而歌，弃衣而走，贲响腹胀，是谓骭厥。是主血所生病者(胃病及血所致的病症)，狂疟温淫，汗出，鼽衄，口㖞，唇胗(口唇生疮)，颈肿，喉痹，大腹水肿，膝膑肿痛，循膺(胸)、乳、气街、股、伏兔、骭(胫骨)外廉、足跗上皆痛，中指(趾)不用。气盛则身以前皆热(前半身皆有热感)。其有余于胃则消谷善饥，溺色黄；气不足，则身以前皆寒栗；胃中寒则胀满。

4) 足太阴脾经

(1)循行

脾足太阴之脉，起于大趾之端(足大趾内侧端，即隐白穴)①，循指内侧白肉际(大趾内侧赤白肉际)，过核骨(第一跖趾关节结

and ascends in front of the medial malleolus[3] to the medial aspect of the calf[4]. It makes its way along the posterior border of the tibia[5], ascends in front of the Liver Channel of Foot-*Jueyin*[6], goes through the anterior medial aspect of the knee and thigh[7], and into the abdominal cavity[8], then enters its pertaining organ, the spleen, and communicates with the stomach[9]. From there it goes through the diaphragm[10], and upwards along the two sides of the throat[11], reaches the root of the tongue and spreads over its lower surface[12],

The branch of the channel sprouts from the stomach, goes upwards through the diaphragm[13], disperses into the heart[14] and connects with the Heart Channel of Hand-*Shaoyin* (See Fig. 4).

(2) Pathological Symptoms

The most obvious symptoms that result from a disorder of the channel itself are as follows: stiff tongue, vomiting after meals, stomachache, flatulence and frequent eructation, which may be alleviated after moving the bowels and breaking wind, and heaviness sensation of the whole body. As for symptoms due to a disorder of the channel affected by disturbance of the spleen, they are mainly in the form of pains in the root of the tongue, akinesia, inappetence, vexation, acute pain in the upper abdomen, loose stool or dysentery, dysuria, jaundice, being unable to lie flat and difficulty in standing, swelling of the medial aspect of the thigh and knee, cold extremities, and disability of the great toe.

5) The Heart Channel of Hand-*Shaoyin*

(1) Course

This channel starts from the heart[1], comes out of the cardiac system (the large vessels connecting with other viscera) and descends through the diaphragm to connect with the small intestine[2].

The branch of the channel sprouts from the cardiac system[3], runs upwards along the side of the throat[4], and joins

节后②，上内踝前廉③，上踹（应作腨，即小腿肚）内④，循胫骨后⑤，交出厥阴（足厥阴肝经）之前⑥，上膝内前廉⑦，入腹⑧，属脾，络胃⑨，上膈⑩，挟咽⑪，连舌本（即舌根），散舌下⑫。

其支者，复从胃别上膈⑬，注心中⑭，交手少阴心经（见图4）。

（2）病症

是动则病舌本强，食则呕，胃脘痛，腹胀善噫，得后与气（解大便、放屁之后），则快然如衰（上述症状减轻），身体皆重。是主脾所生病者，舌本痛（舌根痛），体不能动摇，食不下，烦心，心下急痛，溏瘕泄（大便稀薄或痢疾），水闭（排尿困难），黄疸，不能卧，强立，股膝内肿，厥，足大指（趾）不用。

5）手少阴心经

（1）循行

心手少阴之脉，起于心中①，出属心系（心与其他脏腑相联系之脉），下膈，络小肠②。

其支者，从心系③，上挟咽④，系目系⑤。

the ocular connectors (the structures connectng the eyeball with the brain, including blood vessels and optic nerves)⑤.

The original channel ascends from the cardiac system to the lung and descends to the axilla⑥. And then it travels along the posterior border of the medial aspect of the upper arm, passes behind the Lung Channel of Hand-*Taiyin* and the Pericardium Channel of Hand-*Jueyin*⑦, goes downwards and reaches the cubital fossa. It continues to run along the posterior border of the medial aspect of the forearm⑧, and arrives at the capitate bone proximal to the palm⑨. It travels via the posterior border of the medial aspect of the palm⑩, and then along the medial side of the little finger reaches the tip (Point Shaochong, H 9)⑪, and finally connects with the Small Intestine Channel of Hand-*Taiyang* (See Fig. 5).

(2) Pathological Symptoms

Dry throat, precordial pain and thirst are the most common symptoms resulting from a disorder of the said channel, which is called "*Bijue*" in TCM. A disorder of the channel affected by heart trouble gives rise to icteric sclera, painful hypochondrium and posterior border of the medial aspect of the upper extremities, cold hands and feet, and painful and hot palms.

6) The Small Intestine Channel of Hand-*Taiyang*

(1) Course

This channel starts from the tip of the ulnar side of the little finger (Point Shaoze, SI 1)①, and follows the ulnar border of the dorsum of the hand, ascends to the wrist, and then through the styloid process of the ulna② and the posterior border of the forearm, finally passing between the olecranon of the ulna and the medial epicondyle of the humerus③. It continues to travel along the posterior border of the lateral aspect of the upper arm④, and out of the shoulder joint⑤. Then circling round the shoulder-blade⑥, it meets the *Du* Channel at Point Dazhui (Du 14)⑦. From there it goes forward into the supraclavicular fossa⑧ and then connects with the heart⑨.

其直者，复从心系却上肺，下出腋下[6]，循臑内后廉，行手太阴、心主（手太阴肺经、手厥阴心包经）之后[7]，下肘内，循臂内后廉[8]，抵掌后锐骨之端（掌后豌豆骨部）[9]，入掌内后廉[10]，循小指之内（小指内侧），出其端（少冲穴）[11]，交手太阳小肠经（见图5）。

（2）病症

是动则病嗌干（咽干），心痛，渴而欲饮，是谓臂厥。是主心所生病者，目黄，胁痛，臑臂内后廉痛（上肢内侧后缘痛），厥，掌中热痛。

6）手太阳小肠经

（1）循行

小肠手太阳之脉，起于小指之端（少泽穴）[1]，循手外侧（手背尺侧），上腕，出踝中（尺骨茎突）[2]，直上循臂下廉（前臂后缘）出肘内侧两筋之间（尺骨鹰嘴与肱骨内上髁之间）[3]，上循臑外后廉[4]，出肩解（肩关节）[5]，绕肩胛[6]，交肩上（交会于肩上督脉大椎穴）[7]，入缺盆[8]，络心[9]，循咽（食管）[10]，下膈[11]，抵胃[12]，

cending along the esophagus[10], it passes the diaphragm[11], reaches the stomach[12], and enters its pertaining organ, the small intestine[13].

One of the branches of this channel emerges from the supraclavicular fossa[8], and ascends along the neck[14] to the cheek[16]. From there it reaches the outer canthus of the eye[17], and then goes into the ear (at Point Tinggong, SI 19)[18].

The other branch of the channel, which is separated from the cheek, ascends to the infra-orbital region (Point Quanliao, SI 18), reaches the lateral side of the nose and terminates at the inner canthus[20]. Then it is distributed obliquely over the zygoma[19] and connects with the Urinary Bladder Channel of Foot-*Taiyang* (See Fig. 6).

(3) Pathological Symptoms

The main symptoms due to a disorder of the channel itself are as follows: sore throat, swelling of the chin, stiff neck, unbearable pain in the shoulder as if extracted, and severe pain of the upper arm as if fractured. The primary symptoms which are due to a channel disorder, affected by fluid trouble that is caused by small intestine disease, are shown in the form of deafness, icteric sclera, swelling of the cheek, and pains along the posterior border of the lateral aspect of the neck, the chin, the shoulder, the upper arm, the elbow and the forearm.

7) The Urinary Bladder Channel of Foot-*Taiyang*

(1) Course

This channel commences from the inner canthus[1], ascends to the forehead[2] and joins its symmetrical channel at the vertex (Point Baihui, Du 20)[3].

One of its branches splits off the vertex and goes to the upper aspect of the auricle[4].

The original channel leaves the vertex for the brain[5] where it re-emerges and runs downward to the back of the neck[6]. Continuing along the medial side of the scapula, it

属小肠[13]。

其支者，从缺盆[8]，循颈[14]，上颊[16]，至目锐眦[17]，却入耳中[18]。

其支者，别颊，上䪼（眼眶下部，即颧髎穴），抵鼻（鼻旁），至目内眦[20]，斜络于颧[19]，交足太阳膀胱经（见图6）。

（3）病症

是动则病嗌痛（咽喉痛），颔肿（颏肿），不可以顾（头项不能转侧回顾），肩似拔（肩痛似被拔掉），臑似折（上臂痛如同折断）。是主液所生病者（小肠病及所主之液，进而影响经脉），耳聋，目黄，颊肿，颈、颔、肩、臑、肘、臂外后廉痛。

7）足太阳膀胱经

（1）循行

膀胱足太阳之脉，起于目内眦（眼内角）[1]，上额[2]交巅（百会穴）[3]。

其支者，从巅至耳上角[4]。

其直者，从巅入络脑[5]，还出别下项[6]，循肩髆内（肩胛内

travels parallel to the vertebral column[8] and reaches the lumbar region[8]. Passing the paravertebral muscles[9], it communicates with the kidney[10] and enters into its pertaining organ, the urinary bladder[11].

The branch from the lumbar region runs downwards parallel to the vertebral column (1.5 individual *cun* lateral to the back mid-line), through the gluteal region[12], and into the popliteal fossa[13].

Another branch emerges from the original channel at the back of the neck, from the medial side of the scapula passes through the scapula, and runs downwards parallel to the vertebral column (3 individual *cun* lateral to the back mid-line)[14]. Then it runs through the trochanter major of the femur[15], downwards along the posterior border of the lateral side of the thigh[16] where it meets the branch descending from the lumbar region in the popliteal fossa[17]. From there, it makes its way down through the musculus gastrocnemius[18], emerges from the posterior aspect of the external malleolus[19], runs along Point Jinggu (UB 64)[20] to the lateral side of the tip of the small toe (Point Zhiyin, UB 67)[21], where it connects with the Kidney Channel of Foot-*Shaoyin* (See Fig. 7).

(2) Pathological Symptoms

As a result of a disorder of the channel itself, the patient will have headache with feeling of *qi* rushing upwards, pain in the eyes as if gouged out, pain in the back of the neck as if pulled up, pain in the spine and lumbus as if broken, acampsia of the thigh, spasm of the tendons in the popliteal fossa as if knotted, and pain in the musculus gastrocnemius as if split, which is termed "*Huai Jue*". A patient who suffers from channel disorder that is caused by tendon trouble due to urinary bladder disease will have hemorrhoid, malaria, insanity, epilepsy, icteric sclera, lacrimation, epistaxis, pains in the fontanel and other parts such as the back of the neck, the lumbus, the sacral region, the popliteal fossa, the musculus gastrocnemius, and

侧），挟脊⑦抵腰中⑧，入循膂（脊旁肌肉）⑨，络肾⑩，属膀胱⑪。

其支者，从腰中下挟脊，贯臀⑫，入腘中⑬。

其支者，从膊内左右，别下贯胛，挟脊内⑭，过髀枢（股骨上端的关节部，即大转子）⑮，循髀外（大腿外侧），从后廉（后缘）⑯，下合腘中⑰，以下贯腨（腓肠肌）内⑱，出外踝后⑲，循京骨⑳，至小趾外侧（至阴穴）㉑，交足少阴肾经（见图7）。

（2）病症

是动则病冲头痛，目似脱，项似拔，脊痛，腰似折，髀不可曲（大腿不能弯曲），腘如结，踹如裂（腓肠肌痛如裂），是为踝厥。是主筋所生病者（膀胱病及所主之筋，进而导致该经异常），痔，疟，狂，癫疾，头囟（颇门）项痛，目黄，泪出，鼽衄，项、背、

the foot, and dysfunction of the small toes.

8) The Kidney Channel of Foot-*Shaoyin*

(1) Course

The Kidney Channel of Foot-*Shaoyin* starts from the plantar surface of the little toe, and runs obliquely towards the center of the sole of the foot (Point Yongquan, KI)①. Emerging from Point Rangu (K 2) (at the interior aspect of the tuberosity of the navicular bone)② it runs behind the medial malleolus③, and reaches the heel④. Then it ascends along the medial side of the musculus gastrocnemius⑤ and emerges from the medial side of the popliteal fossa⑥. Ascending continuously along the medio-posterior aspect of the thigh⑦, it runs through the vertebral column. From there it enters its pertaining organ, the kidney⑧, and communicates with the urinary bladder⑨.

Its direct branch re-emerges from the kidney⑩, runs straight up through the liver and diaphragm⑪, into the lung⑫, from which it travels along the throat⑬ and terminates at the root of the tongue⑭.

Another branch of its exits from the lung, connects with the heart, and is distributed over the thoracic cavitys to meet with the Pericardium Channel of Hand-*Jueyin* (See Fig. 8).

(2) Pathological Symptoms

When, due to a disorder of the channel itself, the patient may feel hungry but have no taste for food. In addition, he may have dark complexion, hemoptysis, branchial wheezing, and blurred vision. He may feel uncomfortable when sitting. It seems as if he were so starved that his heart hangs in the air. If this channel is deficient in the *qi* the patient is apt to be nervous and has palpitation with fear of being caught, which is termed "Bone *Jue*". A patient who suffers from channel disorder affected by kidney trouble may have burning sensation of mouth, dry tongue, swollen throat, inspiratory dyspnea,

腰、尻(骶尾部)、腘、踹、脚皆痛，小指(趾)不用。

8)足少阴肾经

(1)循行

肾足少阴之脉，起于小指(趾)之下，斜走足心(涌泉穴)①，出于然谷(位于舟骨粗隆下)②，循内踝之后③，别入跟中④，以上腨内⑤，出腘内廉⑥，上股内后廉⑦，贯脊属肾⑧，络膀胱⑨。

其直者，从肾⑩上贯肝膈⑪，入肺中⑫，循喉咙⑬，挟舌本⑭。

其直者，从肺出络心，注胸中⑮，交手厥阴心包经(见图8)。

(2)病症

是动则病饥不欲食，面如漆柴，咳唾则有血，喝喝而喘，坐而欲起，目䀮䀮(视物不清)，如无所见，心如悬，若饥状。气不足则善恐，心惕惕如人将捕之，是谓骨厥④。是主肾所生病者，

dry sore pharynx, vexation, precordial pain, jaundice, dysentery, pains in the spine and the posterior border of the medial aspect of the thigh, syncope, flaccidity, somnolence, and painful soles with burning sensation.

9) The Pericardium Channel of Hand-*Jueyin*

(1) Course

This channel commences from the chest where it exits from its pertaining organ, the pericardium[1]. Then it descends through the diaphragm[2] and links up with the triple warmers in the upper, the middle and the lower portions of the body cavity[3].

One of its branches runs along the chest[4], through the costal rigion at a point 3 individual *cun* below the armpit[5], and ascends to the axilla[6]. From the medial aspect of the upper arm, it makes its way downwards between the Lung Channel and the Heart Channel[7], and reaches the cubital fossa[8]. From there it runs still further downwards to the forearm between the tendons of m. palmaris longus and m. flexorcarpi[9], and enters the palm[10]. It runs along the middle finger to its tip (Point Zhongchong, P 9)[11].

Another branch of its leaves the palm (Point Laogong, P 8), runs along the ring finger to its tip (Point Guanchong, SJ 1)[12], and connects with the Triple Warmer Channel of Hand-*Shaoyang* (See Fig. 9).

(2) Pathological Symptoms

As result of a disorder of the channel itself the case is symptomatized by feverish sensation in the palm center, spasm and contracture of the arm and elbow, swelling of the axilla, feeling of fullness in the chest and hypochondria, violent palpitation with irritability, flushed face, icteric sclera and mania. If the channel disorder is caused by pericardium trouble, the case is symptomatized by vexation, precordial pain, and hot feeling of the palms.

口热，舌干，咽肿，上气，嗌(咽)干及痛，烦心，心痛，黄疸，肠澼(痢疾)，脊股内后廉痛，痿厥，嗜卧，足下热而痛。

9）手厥阴心包经

（1）循行

心主手厥阴心包络之脉，起于胸中，出属心包络①，下膈②，历络三焦③。

其支者，循胸④出胁，下腋三寸⑤，上抵腋下⑥，循臑内，行太阴、太阴之间⑦，入肘中⑧，下臂，行两筋（掌长肌腱与桡侧腕屈肌腱）之间⑨，入掌中⑩，循中指，出其端(中冲穴)⑪。

其支者，别掌中，循小指次指出其端⑫，交手少阳三焦经(见图9)。

（2）病症

是动则病手心热，臂肘挛急，腋肿，甚则胸胁支满，心中憺憺大动，面赤，目黄，喜笑不休。是主脉所生病者（心包病及其脉所发生的病症)，烦心，心痛，掌中热。

10) The Triple Warmer *Sanjiao* Channel of Hand-*Shaoyang*

(1) Course

The Triple Warmer Channel of Hand-*Shaoyang* starts from the ulnar side of the tip of the ring finger (Point Guanchong, SJ 1)[1], and runs upwards between the two fingers i.e., the 4th and 5th metacarpal bones[2]. Along the dorsum of the wrist[3], it travels to the dorsal side of the forearm between the two bones or the radius and ulna[4]. It goes upwards through the olecranon[5], along the lateral aspect of the upper arm[6], to the shoulder region[7], where it meets the Gall Bladder Channel of Foot-*Shaoyang*, and afterwards leaves its posterior aspect[8] for the supraclavicular fossa[9]. From the fossa it descends further, is distributed to Point Shanzhong (Ren 17), or the region in the centre between the two breasts, and communicates with the pericardium[10]. Descending through the diaphragm, it reaches the triple warmer, i.e. the upper, middle and lower portions of the body cavity in succession[11].

One of its branches originates from Point Shanzhong[12] (Ren 17) and ascends to the supraclavicular fossa[13], from where it goes upwards to the nape of the neck[14]. From the posterior border of the ear[15], it makes a direct ascent through the superior aspect of the auricula[16], curves down the cheek, and then rea ches the infraorbital region[17].

Another branch originates in the retro-auricular region and passes into the ear. Emerging in front of the ear, it runs in front of Kezhuren, i.e.,Point Shangguan (GB 3), acrosses the above-mentioned branch at the cheek[18] and reaches the outer canthus[19], where it connects with the Gall Bladder Channel of Foot-*Shaoyang* (See Fig. 10).

(2) Pathological Symptoms

Symptoms due to a disorder of the channel itself are as follows: deafness, tinnitus, swelling of the pharynx and sore

10）手少阳三焦经

（1）循行

三焦手少阳之脉，起于小指次指之端（即无名指尺侧端之关冲穴）[1]，上出两指之间（即第四、五掌骨之间）[2]，循手表腕（腕背）[3]，出臂外两骨之间（即前臂外侧桡骨和尺骨之间）[4]，上贯肘（尖）[5]，循臑外[6]，上肩[7]而交出足少阳（胆经）之后[8]，入缺盆[9]，布膻中，散络心包[10]，下膈，循属三焦[11]。

其支者，从膻中[12]，上出缺盆[13]，上项[14]，系耳后，直上[15]，出耳上角[16]，以屈下颊至䪼（由此弯曲下行至眼眶下部）[17]。

其支者，从耳后，入耳中，出走耳前，过客主人（上关穴）前，交颊[18]，至目锐眦[19]，交足少阳胆经（见图10）。

（2）病症

是动则病耳聋，浑浑焞焞（耳鸣），嗌肿，喉痹。是主气所生

throat. A channel disorder that is caused when its *qi* is troubled, or when its relevant organ is diseased,has the following manifestations: hidrosis, pain in the outer canthus of the eye, pain in the cheek pains in the posterior border of the ear and along the lateral aspect of the shoulder, upper arm, elbow and forearm, and dysfunction of the ring finger.

11) The Gall Bladder Channel of Foot-*Shaoyang*

(1) Course

This channel starts from the outer canthus of the eye[1], runs upwards to the corner of the forehead[2], and curves downwards to the retro-auricular region[3]. Then it runs along the side of the neck in front of the Triple Warmer Channel[4] to the shoulder. Turning backwards it goes behind the Triple Warmer Channel of Hand-*Shaoyang*, and enters the supraclavicular fossa[5].

One of its branches originates in the retro-auricular region, passes through the ear[6], re-emerges in front of the ear[7] and then reaches the posterior aspect of the outer canthus of the eye[8].

Another branch leaves the outer canthus[9] for Point Daying (St 5)[10]. and meets the Triple Warmer Channel of Hand-*Shaoyang* again. From there it reaches the infraorbital region[11], thendescends through Point Jiache(St 6)[12] to the neck, from where it passes into the supraclavicular fossa and meets the original channel[13]. Then it continues to travel through the chest, the diaphragm[14], the liver[15], and then to the gall bladder[16]. It then travels along the inside of the hypochondrium[17], through Point Qijie or Qichong (St 30)[18], around the margin of the pubisure[19], transversely into Point Huantiao (GB 30)[20].

A third straight branch descends from the supraclavicular fossa[21] to the axilla[22], from where it continues its descent along

病者，汗出，目锐眦(外眼角)痛，颊痛，耳后、肩、臑、肘、臂外皆痛，小指次指(小指侧的第二指，即无名指)不用。

11)足少阳胆经

(1)循行

胆足少阳之脉，起于目锐眦(眼外角)①，上抵头角(额角)②，下耳后③，循颈行手少阳(三焦经)之前④，至肩上却交出手少阳之后，入缺盆⑤。

其支者，从耳后入耳中⑥，出走耳前⑦，至目锐眦后⑧。

其支者，别锐眦⑨，下大迎⑩，合于手少阳，抵于䪼(目眶下部)⑪，下加颊车⑫，下颈，合缺盆⑬。以下胸中，贯膈⑭，络肝⑮，属胆⑯，循胁里⑰，出气街⑱，绕毛际⑲，横入髀厌中(环跳穴)⑳。

其直者，从缺盆㉑，下腋㉒，循胸㉓，过季胁㉔，下合髀厌

the lateral aspect of the chest[23], through the hypochondrium[24], to Huantiao(GB 30), and meets the above-mentioned branch[25]. From Huantiao(GB 30), it goes down along the lateral aspect of the thigh[26], emerges from the lateral side of the knee[27], and continues its downward travel along the anterior aspect of the fibula[28], and straight to *Juegu*, i.e. a hollow in the low part of the fibula and 3 individual *cun* above the external malleolus[29]. Running further downwards, it emerges in front of the external malleolus. Along the dorsum of the foot[30], it finds its terminus at the lateral side of the tip of the 4th toe[31].

A fourth branch leaves the dorsum of the foot, makes its way first between the lst and 2nd metatarsal bones, then through the distal portion of the big toe, back to its nail and finally out of the hair portion proximal to it[32], and communicates with the Liver Channel of Foot-*Jueyin* (See Fig. 11).

(2) Pathological Symptoms

A patient who suffers from a disorder of the channel itself may have the following symptoms: bitter taste, frequent sighing, precordial and hypochondriac pains, unable to turn round, sallow complexion (in serious cases), asteatosis cutis, and hot feeling of the lateral aspect of the dorsum of the foot, which is called "*Yang Jue*" in TCM. A patien twho suffers from bone disorder caused by gall bladder trouble may have headache, pains in the chin, in the outer canthus of the eye, and in the supraclavicular fossa, edema of the axilla, tuberculosis of the lymph nodes, hidrosis, shivering, malaria, and pains along the course of this channel such as the chest, hypochondrium, rib, thigh, lateral aspect of the part from knee to fibula and its lower part, external malleolus and joints, and dysfunction of the 4th toe.

12) The Liver Channel of Foot-*Jueyin*

(1) Course

The Liver Channel of Foot-*Jueyin* starts from the border

中㉕，以下循髀阳(大腿外侧)㉖，出膝外廉㉗，下外辅骨之前(腓骨前面)㉘，直下，抵绝骨之端（腓骨下段，外踝上三寸之陷凹处)㉙，下出外踝之前，循足跗(足背)上㉚，入小趾次趾之间(足第四趾外侧端)㉛。

其支者，别跗上，入大趾之间，循大趾歧骨内，出其端，还贯爪甲，出三毛㉜，交足厥阴肝经(见图11)。

(2)病症

是动则病口苦，善太息，心胁痛，不能转侧，甚则面有微尘，体无膏泽，足外反热，是为阳厥。是主骨所生病者，头痛，颔痛，目锐眦痛，缺盆中肿痛，腋下肿，马刀侠瘿，汗出，振寒，疟，胸、胁、髀(股)、膝外至胫、绝骨、外踝前及诸节皆痛，小指次指不用。

12)足厥阴肝经

(1)循行

of the hair behind the nail of the great toe[1], passes the dorsum of the foot[2] and reaches the region one individual *cun* in front of the medial malleolus[3]. From there, it ascends 8 individual *cun* above the medial malleolus where it crosses the Spleen Channel of Foot-*Taiyin*, then runs behind the channel[4] up to the medial border of the popliteal fossa[5]. It continues its ascent along the medial side of the thigh[6], to the pubic region[7] where it curves round the external genitalia[8] and enters the lower abdomen[9]. From there, it runs upwards via the stomach into its pertaining organ, the liver, and communicates with the gall bladder[10]. Further upward, it passes through the diaphragm[11], is distributed to the hypochondrium[12], and ascends along the posterior aspect of the larynx[13] to the nasopharynx[14], where it connects with the surrounding tissues of the eye[15], then emerges from the forehead[16], and finally meets the *Du* Channel at the vertex[17].

One of its branches originates in the tissues connecting the eye ball with the brain, goes downwards into the cheek[18] and curves round the inner surface of the lips[19].

Another branch originates in the liver[20], passes through the diaphragm[21] and penetrates to the lung[22], where it connects with the Lung Channel of Hand-*Taiyin* (See Fig. 12).

(2) Pathological Symptoms

If the case results from a disorder of the channel itself, it is symptomatized by lumbago which prevents the patient from bending, swollen painful testes, edema of the lower abdomen in females, dry throat in serious cases and sallow complexion. If the case is due to a channel disorder affected by liver trouble, it is manifested as feeling of fullness in the chest, vomiting, watery diarrhea containing undigested food, inguinal hernia, bed-wetting and dysuria.

肝足厥阴之脉，起于大趾丛毛之际[1]，上循足跗上廉[2]，去内踝一寸（内踝前一寸）[3]，上踝八寸（内踝上八寸），交出太阴之后[4]，上腘内廉[5]，循股阴（股部内侧）[6]，入毛中[7]，过阴器[8]，抵小腹[9]，挟胃，属肝络胆[10]，上贯膈[11]，布胁肋[12]，循喉咙之后[13]，上入颃颡（鼻咽部）[14]，连目系[15]，上出额[16]，与督脉会于巅[17]。

其支者，从目系，下颊里[18]，环唇内[19]。

其支者，复从肝[20]，别贯膈[21]，上注肺[22]，交手太阴肺经（见图12）。

（2）病症

是动则病腰痛不可俯仰，丈夫㿉疝，妇人少腹肿，甚则嗌干，面尘脱色。是主肝所生病者，胸满，呕逆，飧泄（完谷不化的腹泻），狐疝，遗尿，闭癃。

3. The Law Governing the Course, Direction, Joint of the Twelve Channels

The three *yin* channels of the hand travel from the chest to the hand where they join the three *yang* channels of the hand. The three *yang* channels of the hand ascend from the hand to the head where they connect with the three *yang* channels of the foot. The three *yang* channels of the foot descend from the head to the foot where they meet with the three *yin* channels of the foot. The three *yin* channels of the foot ascend from the foot to the abdomen (or chest) where they join the three *yin* channels of the hand. Thus the Twelve Channels form a circulatory path by which the *yin* and *yang* are linked with each other, like an endless ring. This is the law governing the course, direction and joining of the Twelve Channels.

4. The Distributing Law of the Twelve Channels

The distributing law of the Twelve Channels is: In the region of the head and face, the Channels of Hand-*Taiyang* and Foot-*Taiyang* run through both sides of the head, while the Channels of Hand-*Yangming* and Foot-*Yangming* run through the face and forehead. The Channels of Hand-*Taiyang* and Foot-*Taiyang* run through the cheek, the vertex and the back of the neck. In the region of the trunk, the three *yang* channels of the hand run through the shoulder. Of the three *yang* channels of the foot, the *Yangming* runs in front of the trunk (the ventral aspect), the *Taiyang* along the back (the dorsal aspect), and the *Shaoyang* along the sides. All three *yin* channels of the hand exit from the axilla without exception. All three *yin* channels of the foot run through the surface of the abdomen. The channels running through the surface of the abdomen are termed Foot-*Shaoyin*, Foot-*Yangming*, Foot-*Taiyin*, Foot-*Jueyin* in order of their distribution from inside to outside. The law

3. 十二经脉的走向与交接规律

十二经脉的走向、交接规律是：手三阴经，从胸走手，交手三阳经；手三阳经，从手走头，交足三阳经；足三阳经，从头走足，交足三阴经；足三阴经，从足走腹(或胸)，交手三阴经。这样，就构成了"阴阳相贯、如环无端"的循环径路。

4. 十二经脉的分布规律

十二经脉在体表的分布规律是：在头部、面部，手、足太阳经行于侧部，手、足阳明经行于面部、额部，手、足太阳经行于面颊、头项及头后部；在躯干部，手三阳经行于肩胛部，足三阳经，则阳明行于前(腹面)，太阳行于后(背面)，少阳行于侧面。手三阴经均从腋下走出，足三阴经均行于腹面。循行于腹面的经脉，按其自内向外的顺序是足少阴、足阳明、足太阴、足厥阴。十二

governing the distribution of the Twelve Channels in the extremities is shown in the caption below the table "Classification of the Twelve Channels".

5. The Exterior-Interior Relationship between the Twelve Channels

The Twelve Channels are linked with each other through the internal branches and the reticular branches, which constitute six pairs of exterior-interior relationship. Please see the following list:

Exterior-interior Relationship of the Twelve Channels

(1) The exterior-interior-relationship between the Small Intestine Channel of Hand-*Taiyang* and the Heart Channel of Hand-*Shaoyin*
(2) The exterior-interior-relationship between the Triple Warmer Channel of Hand-*Shaoyang* and the Pericardium Channel of Hand-*Jueyin*
(3) The exterior-interior-relationship between the Large Intestine Channel of Hand-*Yangming* and the Lung Channel of Hand-*Taiyin*
(4) The exterior-interior-relationship between the Urinary Bladder Channel of Foot-*Taiyang* and the Kidney Channel of Foot-*Shaoyin*
(5) The exterior-interior-relationship between the Gall Bladder Channel of Foot-*Shaoyang* and the Liver Channel of Foot-*Jueyin*
(6) The exterior-interior-relationship between the Stomach Channel of Foot-*Yangming* and the Spleen Channel of Foot-*Taiyin*

Note:

The two channels with the exterior-interior relation run along the opposite regions of both sides of the extremities (but the Liver Channel of Foot-*Jueyin* and the Spleen Channel of Foot-*Taiyin* shift their positions in the region 8 individual *cun* above the medial malleolus). They join each other at the hand or the foot.

The exterior-interior relations of the Twelve Channels not only strengthen the connection between the exterior channels and the interior channels, coordinate the viscera and bowels that are of mutual exterior-interior relationship in terms of physiology, but also cause them to have a pathological influence on each other. In treatment, acupuncture points of the channels with mutual exterior-interior re-

经脉在四肢的分布规律，可参见“十二经脉之分类”表下面的解释。

5．十二经脉的表里关系

十二经脉通过经别和别络互相沟通，组合成六对表里相合关系，见下表：

十二经脉的表里关系

十二经脉的表里关系
（1）手太阳小肠经与手少阴心经相表里
（2）手少阳三焦经与手厥阴心包经相表里
（3）手阳明大肠经与手太阴肺经相表里
（4）足太阳膀胱经与足少阴肾经相表里
（5）足少阳胆经与足厥阴肝经相表里
（6）足阳明胃经与足太阴脾经相表里

注：凡有表里关系的经脉，均行于四肢两个侧面的相对部位（足厥阴肝经与足太阴脾经在内踝上八寸处交叉变换位置），并在手或足相互交换。

十二经脉的表里关系，不仅加强了表里两经的联系，而且使相为表里的脏腑在生理上得以相互配合，在病理上亦相互影响。在

lationship can be alternatively used. For example, in treating disease of the large intestine, one can use the point of the Lung Channel of Hand-*Taiyin*. Its theoretical basis can be found from above.

6. The Flowing Order of the Twelve Channels

The motion of the "*qi*" and blood inside the Twelve Channels is circulative and continuous. The "*qi*" and blood start their circulation from the Lung Channel of Hand-*Taiyin*, then pass through the last channel, the Liver Channel of Foot-*Jueyin*, and again to the Lung Channel of Hand-*Taiyin*. The terminus of one channel connects with the starting point of another channel, thus forming an endless ring. See the following table:

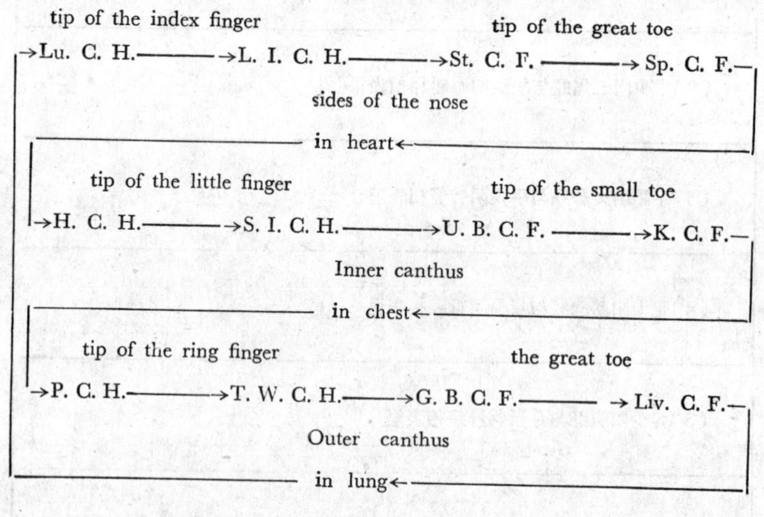

Section 3

The Eight Extra Channels

"The Eight Extra Channels" is a general term for the *Du*, *Ren*, *Chong*, *Dai*, *Yinqiao*, *Yangqiao*, *Yinwei* and *Yangwei* Channels. They are called "the Eight Extra Channels" because

治疗上，相为表里的两条经脉的俞穴可以交叉使用。如治疗大肠病，可取肺经穴。其理论根据，即源于此。

6. 十二经脉的流注次序

十二经脉中的气血运行，是循环贯注的。即从手太阴肺经开始，依次传至足厥阴肝经，然后再传手太阴肺经，首尾相贯，如环无端。见下表：

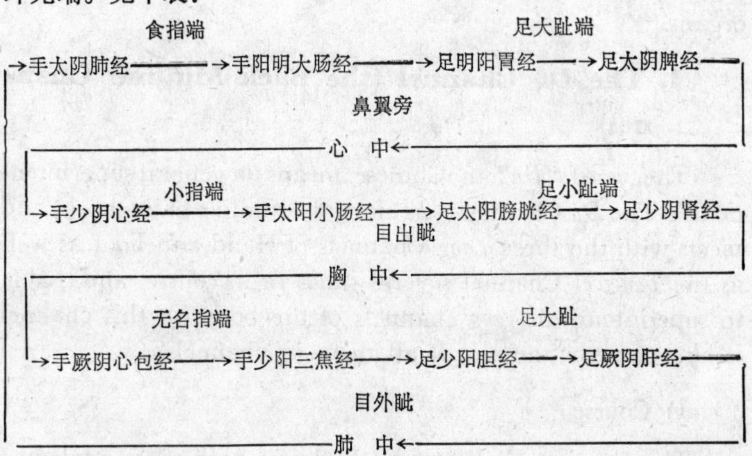

第三节 奇经八脉

奇经八脉是督脉、任脉、冲脉、带脉、阴跷脉、阳跷脉、阴

their courses are not as regular as those of the above-mentioned Twelve Channels, because they have no direct relationship with any of the internal organs, or exterior-interior coordination between them and because their total number is eitht.

The Eight Extra Channels crisscross the regular twelve channels, and perform the functions of strengthening the ties between the channels and regulating the "*qi*" and blood inside the twelve regular channels. When the blood and *qi* inside the Twelve Channels are full and overflowing, the excess will be stored in the Eight Extra Channels. On the other hand when those are insufficient, they will be supplemented from the Eight Extra Channels. The Eight Extra Channels are not only more closely related to the liver, kidney and other internal organs, but also to the uterus, brain, marrow and extra ordinary organs.

1. The *Du* Channel (the Back Midline Channel)

The word "*Du*" in Chinese means "a general superintendent". The *Du* Channel runs along the midline of the back, and meets with the three *Yang* Channels of Hand and Foot as well as the *Yangwei* Channel several times in its course, and is able to superintend all *yang* channels of the body, so this channel is also named "the sea of all the *yang* channels".

1) Course

The channel originates in the lower part of the abdomen below the umbilicus, makes its downward way through the perineum ①, then ascends along the middle of the spinal column②, and reaches Dulb Fengfu at the back of the neck where it enters the brain③. It continues to ascend from Fengfu (Du 16), along the midline of the head and passing the vertex④, forehead, columella of the nose and the upper lip, then to Yinjiao (Du 28) (See Fig. 13).

维脉和阳维脉的总称。由于它们的循行不象十二经脉那样规则，与脏腑无直接的“络属”关系，彼此之间亦无表里配合，且其脉有八，故称“奇经八脉”。

奇经八脉纵横交叉于十二经脉之间，具有加强经脉之间的联系、调节正经气血的作用。当十二经脉中的气血满溢时，就流蓄于奇经八脉；不足时，则由奇经八脉予以补充。奇经八脉与肝、肾等脏以及女子胞、脑、髓等奇恒之腑，关系较为密切。

1.督脉

督，在汉语里有“总管”之意。督脉行于背部正中，多次与手、足三阳经及阳维脉交会，能总督一身之阳经，故又称“阳脉之海”。

1)循行

督脉起于小腹内，下出会阴①，沿脊柱正中上行②，至项后风府穴进入脑内③，再由风府穴沿头部正中线上行，经头顶④、

The branches from this channel connect with the kidney and travel through the heart.

2) Pathological Symptoms

Rigid spine, opisthotonus, rachialgia, dorsalgia, headache, insanity, emission of sperm, impotence, premature ejaculation, sterility, prolapse of rectum, etc.

2. The *Ren* (the Front Midline) Channel

The word "*Ren*" in Chinese means "take charge". The *Ren* Channel runs along the midline of the venter, meets with the three *Yin* Channels of the Hand and Foot as well as the *Yinwei* Channel many times in its course, and takes charge of all the *yin* channels of the whole body, so it is also named "the sea of all the *yin* channels". In addition, as the *Ren* Channel is related to pregnancy, there is a way of saying it, "the *Ren* Channel is in charge of pregnancy".

1) Course

This channel originates in the uterus, and makes its downward way through the perineum①, across the pubisure part②, along the midline of the abdomen and the chest③, through the throat④ to the mandible where it turns round the lips and up to Yinjiao (Du 28)⑤. Via the face⑥, two branches of the channel ascend to the regions below the orbits of the eyes⑦ (See Fig. 14).

2) Pathological Symptoms

Menoxenia, sterility, abortion, profuse leukorrhea, hernia, mass in the abdomen, sore throat, etc.

3. The *Chong* Channel (the Vital Channel)

The *Chong* Channel controls and regulates the "*qi*" and blood inside the twelve regular channels, so it is named "the

额部、鼻部、上唇，至龈交穴[5]（见图13）。有支脉络肾、贯心。

2）病症

脊柱强直，角弓反张，脊背痛，头痛，精神失常，遗精，阳痿，早泄，不育，脱肛等。

2.任脉

任，在汉语里有"担任"之意。任脉行于腹面正中线，多次与手、足三阴经及阴维脉交会，能总任一身之阴经，故又称"阴脉之海"。此外，由于任脉与妊娠有关，故有"任主胞胎"之说。

1）循行

任脉起于胞中，下出会阴[1]，向前进入阴毛部[2]，沿腹、胸正中线上行[3]，通过咽喉[4]，到达下颌，环绕口唇，上至龈交[5]，经过面部[6]，分行至目眶下[7]（见图 14）。

2）病症

月经不调，不育，流产，带下，疝气，腹内包块，咽喉疼痛等。

3.冲脉

冲脉有总领、调节十二经脉气血的作用，故有"十二经 脉之

sea of the Twelve Channels" or "the sea of blood". This channel is closely related to the menses.

1) Course

This channel originates in the uterns, descends and emerges at the perineum[1], then ascends through the spinal column[2]. The superficial branch of the channel passes Point Qichong (St 30), meets with the Kidney Channel of Foot-*Shaoyin*, and runs along the both sides of the abdomen, reaches the throat and finally goes round the lips[5] (See Fig. 15),

2) Pathological Symptoms

Menstrual disorder, uterine bleeding, sterility, hypogalactia, spitting blood, abnormal rising of *qi*, spasm in abdomen, etc.

4. The *Dai* Channel (the Belt Channel)

The word "*Dai*" in Chinese means "a belt". The *Dai* Channel runs transversely round the waist like a belt. That is why it is termed the *Dai* Channel (the Belt Channel). It binds all the channels of the body, fixing and safeguarding the foetus and controling the secretion of the leucorrhea.

1) Course

This channel starts below the hypochondrium, descends obliguely to Point Daimai (GB 26)[1], then runs transveresly round the waist[2] (See Fig. 16).

2) Pathological Symptoms

Profuse leucorrhea, abortion, hysteroptosis, abdominal distention, soreness and debility of the waist, etc.

5. The *Yinqiao* Channel and the *Yangqiao* Channel

"*Qiao*" in Chinese means "nimble". The *Yangqiao* Chan-

海”、“血海”之称。冲脉与月经密切相关。

1)循行

冲脉起于胞中，下出会阴①，向上行于脊柱之内②；其外行者，经气冲与足少阴肾经交会，沿腹部两侧③，上达咽喉④，环绕口唇⑤(见图15)。

2)病症

月经不调，崩漏，不育，乳少，吐血，逆气里急等。

4.带脉

带，在汉语里有“束带”之意。带脉围腰一周，状如束带，故名带脉。它具有约束诸脉、固护胎儿和主司妇女带下的作用。

1)循行

带脉起于季胁之下，斜向下行至带脉穴①，绕身一周②(见图16)。

2)病症

带下，流产，子宫脱垂，腹部胀满，腰酸无力等。

5.阴跷脉、阳跷脉

跷，在汉语里有“轻健跷捷”之意。阳跷脉能主一身左右之

nel can control the "*yang*" of the left and right sides of the whole body, while the *Yinqiao* Channel not only controls the "*yin*" of the left and right sides of the whole body, but also nourishes the eyes, controls the opening and closing of the eyelids as well as the motion of the lower limbs.

1) Course

The *Qiao* Channels are made up of the *Yinqiao* and *Yangqiao* Channels, both of which originate in the region below the malleoli, but run separately along the left and right sides of the body.

The *Yinqiao* Channel ascends from Point Zhaohai (K 6) below the medial malleolus① to the upper portion of the malleolus②. Then it runs along the medio-posterior aspect of the lower limbs③, straight to the external genitalia④. From there it ascends further along the abdomen and chest⑤ into the supraclavicular fossa⑥. Running along the throat, it passes in front of Point Renying (St 9)⑦ and the medial side of the zygomatic region⑧, and reaches the inner canthus of the eye where the channel meets with the *Taiyang* Channels of Hand and Foot as well as the *Yangqiao* Channel (See Fig. 17)⑨.

The *Yangqiao* Channel travels from Shenmai (UB 62) below the external malleolus,① up to the malleolus, through the posterior border of the fibula② and the lateral side of the thigh, to the posterior aspect of the hypochondriac region. Via the posterior axillary fold, it winds its way through the shoulder and ascends along the neck to the corner of the mouth. Passing the side of the naris, it goes into the inner canthus where the channel communicates with the *Taiyang* Channels of the Hand and Foot as well as the *Yinqiao* Channel. From there it travels along the Urinary Bladder Channel of Foot-*Taiyang* to the forehead upward into the hairline, then goes behind the ear and meets with the Gall Bladder Channel of Foot-*Shaoyang* at Point Fengchi (GB 20)③ (See Fig. 18).

阳，阴跷脉不仅主一身左右之阴，并能濡养眼目，主司眼睑开合和下肢运动。

1)循行

跷脉左右成对，阴阳跷脉均起于足踝下。

阴跷脉起于内踝下照海穴①，上行于内踝的上部②，沿下肢内侧后缘直上③，至前阴部④，再上沿腹、胸部⑤，进入缺盆⑥，沿喉咙出人迎穴之前⑦，经颧骨部内侧⑧，至目内眦，与手足太阳经和阳跷脉会合⑨（见图17）。

阳跷脉起于外踝下申脉穴①，沿外踝上行，经腓骨后缘②、大腿外侧，至胁肋后方，从腋缝后上肩，沿颈部上挟口角，经鼻孔旁，至目内眦，与手、足太阳经和阴跷脉会合，再沿足太阳膀胱经上额，入发际，循行至耳后，与足少阳胆经会于风池穴③（见图18）。

2) Pathological Symptoms

Yinqiao disease is symptomatized by myasthenia of the lateral side of the limbs and myospasm of the medial side of the limbs, laryngalgia and somnolence. *Yangqiao* disease is symptomatized by myasthenia of the medial side of the limbs and myospasm of the lateral side of the limbs, insanity, insomnia and pain in the inner canthus.

6. The *Yinwei* Channel and the *Yangwei* Channel

"*Wei*" in Chinese means "maintain and communicate". The *Yinwei* Channel serves to maintain and communicate with all the *yin* channels of the body, while the *Yangwei* Channel serves all the *yang* channels.

1) Course

The *Yinwei* Channel originates in the region where three *yin* channels cross at the medial aspect of the calf[1], ascends along the medial aspect of the lower extremities and reaches the abdomen[2] to join the Spleen Channel of Foot-*Taiyin*[3]. From there it runs upward to the hypochondrium to meet with the Liver Channel of Foot-*Jueyin*. Then it ascends along the chest[4] to communicate with the *Ren* Channel at the neck[5] (See Fig. 19).

The *Yangwei* Channel originates in the heel[1], exits from the external malleouls[2] and ascends along the course of the Gall Bladder Channel of Foot-*Shaoyang*. It passes the lateral aspect of the lower extremity[3] and lateral-posterior side of the trunk[4], ascends behind the axilla to the shoulder[5]. From there it continues its travel through the neck towards the forehead[6], spreading over the sides of the head and the back of the neck and thus communicating with the *Du* Channel[7] (See Fig. 20).

2）病症

阴跷为病，肢体外侧肌肉弛缓而内侧肌肉拘急，喉痛，嗜睡；阳跷为病，肢体内侧肌肉弛缓而外侧拘急，癫狂，失眠，目内眦痛。

6. 阴维脉、阳维脉

维，在汉语有“维系”之意。阴维脉的功能是维络诸阴经；阳维脉则是维络诸阳经。

1）循行

阴维脉起于小腿内侧足三阴经交会之处①，沿下肢内侧上行至腹部②，与足太阴脾经相合③，至胁部，与足厥阴肝经相合，然后沿胸部上行④，与任脉会于颈部⑤（见图 19）。

阳维脉起于足跟部①，向上出于外踝②，沿足少阳胆经上行，经下肢外侧③、躯干后外侧④，从腋后上肩⑤，经颈部，到前额⑥，分布于头侧及项后，与督脉会合⑦（见图 20）。

2) Pathological Symptoms

Disturbance of the *Yinwei* Channel gives rise to the following symptoms: chest pain, stomachache and precordial pain. Disturbance of the *Yangwei* Channel causes symptoms such as alternate spells of chill and fever.

Section 4

The Physiology and Application of the Channels and Collaterals

1. The Physiological Functions of the Chan nels and Collaterals

The physiological function of the channels is known as "the channel *qi*" in TCM. In this section, we shall be concerned with their main physiological functions.

1) Connecting All Parts of the Whole Body

The human body consists of the five viscera, six bowels, five sense organs, skin, muscles, tendons, bones, etc. Each of them has its own special physiological function. It is through the connecting role of the channels that these functions can be coordinated, thus making the body an organic whole.

2) Transporting the *Qi* and Blood To Nourish the Whole Body

Only by receiving nourishment from the "*qi*" and blood can each of the organs in the body give full play to its physiological functions. Most importantly, the channels are the passage-way through which the "*qi*" and blood circulate. ***Classic on Medical Problems*** states, "The function of the channel is to

2）病症

阴维脉为病，表现为胸痛、胃痛、心痛等；阳维脉为病，多为寒热反复发作等。

第四节　经络的生理与应用

1. 经络的生理功能

中医把经络的生理功能称为“经气”。现将其主要生理功能分述如下：

1）联系全身各部

人体由五脏六腑、四肢百骸、五官九窍及皮、肉、筋、骨等组成，它们各有其独特的生理功能。只有通过经络的联系作用，这些功能才能达到相互配合、相互协调，从而使人体形成一个有机的整体。

2）输送气血，濡养全身

人体的各个脏器，只有得到气血的濡养，才能发挥其正常的生理功能。而经络正是气血运行的道路，如《难经》说：“经脉者，

transport the *qi* and blood and circulate *yin* and *yang* in order to nourish the body.

3) Induction, Transmission and Regulation

The channels induce stimulation and transmit information. If some region of the human body is stimulated, such stimulation will be transmitted along the channel to the related viscera or bowels in the body. As a result, the relevant physiological or pathological changes take place. These changes are reflected on the body surface through the channels. "Getting the *qi*" and "circulating the *qi*", the normal sensation felt by the patient during acupuncture, truly embody the inducing and transmitting functions of the channels and collaterals.

The channels and collaterals can regulate the functional activities of the human body, keeping them coordinated and balanced. When dysfunction occurs in some organ, acupuncture and other therapy can be used in order to help further stimulate the regulating function of the channels, and bring the organ back to normality. For example, experiments have proved that it can regulate peristalsis and secretion of the stomach to puncture Zusanli (St 36) of the Stomach Channel of Foot-*Yangming*. When deficiency occurs in peristalses and secretion of the stomach, stimulating this point gently with a needle may strengthen the peristalses of the stomach and increase gastric acidity; if peristalses and secretion of the stomach are excessive, a forceful stimulation in the point with a needle will have an inhibitory effect. Another example, puncturing Neiguan, (P 6) of the Pericardium Channel of Hand-*Jueyin* can cure both bradycardia and tachycardia, performing a diphasic regulative function.

行血气，通阴阳，以荣于身者也。”

3）感应、传导调节

经络有感应刺激、传导信息的作用。当人体的某一部位受到刺激时，这个刺激就可沿着经脉传入体内有关脏腑，使其发生相应的生理或病理变化。而这些变化，又可通过经络反应于体表。针刺中的“得气”、“行气”，就是经络感应、传导功能的具体体现。

经络能调节人体的机能活动，使之保持协调、平衡。当人体的某一脏器功能异常时，可运用针刺等治疗方法来进一步激发经络的调节功能，从而使功能异常的脏器恢复正常。例如，某些试验证明，针刺足阳明胃经的足三里穴可调节胃的蠕动与分泌。当胃的蠕动与分泌呈现不足时，轻刺激该穴，可使胃蠕动增加，胃酸增加；而当胃的蠕动与分泌处于亢奋状态时，强刺激该穴，却引起抑制性效应。再如针刺手厥阴心包经的内关穴，既可治疗心动过缓，又可治疗心动过速，呈双向调节作用。

2. The Application of the Theory of the Channels and Collaterals

1) Explaining Pathological Changes

The channels and collaterals have a direct bearing on the occurence and progress of diseases. If a channel is in functional disorder, it is apt to be attacked by exogenous factors; then the exogenous factors will further intrude into the internal organs along the channels.

The channels and collaterals are not only the route along which exogenous factors intrude into the internal organs from the body surface, but also the way through which the pathological changes between the viscera, and between the internal organs and the tissues of the body surface affect one another. For instance, just as the Liver Channel of Foot-*Jueyin* runs by the stomach and pours into the lung, so liver disease may affect the stomach or lung; owing to the fact that the Kidney Channel of Foot-*Shaoyin* enters the lung and connects with the heart, the retention of fluid, which is due to kidney-asthenia, may attack the lung or heart; and because the Heart Channel of Hand-*Shaoyin* runs along the posterior border of the medial aspect of the upper arm, angina pectoris often radiates to the region.

2) Helping Diagnose Diseases

As the channels differ in their running courses and pertaining organs, during the diagnosis an inference about the channel or organ where pathological changes take place can be drawn from the analysis of where symptoms and signs are located. For example, pains in the hypochondrium probably indicate that the trouble lies in the liver or gall bladder because the hypochondrium is the region where travel Liver Channel of Foot-*Jueyin* and the Gallbladder Channel of Foot-*Shaoyang*; pains in the supraclavicular fossa are mostly caused by lung disease because the supraclavicular fossa is the place where the

2. 经络学说的应用

1）解释病理变化

经络与疾病的发生、传变密切相关。某一经络功能异常，就易遭受外邪的侵袭；既病之后，外邪又可沿着经络进一步内传脏腑。

经络不仅是外邪由表入里的传变途径，而且也是内脏之间、内脏与体表组织之间病变相互影响的途径。如足厥阴肝经挟胃、注肺中，故肝病可以犯胃、犯肺；足少阴肾经入肺、络心，故肾虚水泛可以凌心、射肺；手少阴心经行于上肢内侧后缘，故真心痛常放射至这些部位。

2）协助疾病诊断

由于经络的循行部位不同，所属脏腑各异，故诊断时可通过分析症状出现的部位，来推断病变所在的经络、脏腑。例如：胁部疼痛，多病在肝胆，因胁部是足厥阴肝经和足少阳胆经的循行之处；缺盆中痛，多病变在肺，因缺盆乃手太阴肺经所过之处。再如头痛，可根据经络在头部的分花规律进行诊断，即前额痛多属

Lung Channel of Hand-*taiyin* passes. Another example, headache may be diagnosed in the light of the distributing law of the channels on the head because the pain in the forehead is most probably caused by *Yangming* Channel disturbance; migraine by *Shaoyang* Channel disturbance; pains of the back of the head and neck by *Taiyang* Channel disturbance and pain of the top of the head by *Jueyin* Channel disturbance. In recent years, people have also found that tenderness may occur at Point Zhongfu (L 1) in case of lung disease, at Point Lanwei (Extra 37) in case of acute appendicitis, etc. All these discoveries are helpful in diagnosis.

3) Directing Clinical Treatment

The theory of the channels and collaterals has long been widely applied to direct clinical treatment of all the departments of TCM, in particular, acupuncture, moxibustion, massage and herbal prescriptions. For instance, "the method of selecting points along the channels" is a good example. To be more specific, Point Zusanli (S 36) of the Stomach Chan nel of Foot-*Jangming* should be selected for the treatment of stomachache; Point Qimen (Liv 14) of the Liver Channel Foot-*Jueyin* should be punctured for curing liver disease. The selection of regions of massage is also based on this theory.

It is also through the channels and collaterals that the herbs exert an influence on the pathological region and take effect as expected. Through protracted and repeated practice, TCM doctors have discovered that a certain herb posseses a selective effect for a certain disease of some channel and its pertaining organ, thus creatively formulating a theory of "classifying herbs according to their respective therapeutic effect on the disease of a specific channel and its pertaining organ". For example, through the work done by Chinese ephedra (*Herba Ephedrae*) on the channels of the lung and urinary bladder, sweat is induced, asthma relieved, and diuresis promoted.

阳明，偏头痛多属少阳，头项痛多属太阳，头顶痛多属厥阴。近年来，人们还发现，肺脏有病，中府穴可有压痛；急性阑尾炎，在阑尾穴可有压痛等。这些均有助于疾病的诊断。

3）临床治疗指导

经络学说早已被广泛应用于指导临床各科的治疗，特别是针灸、按摩和中药处方。如针灸中的“循经取穴法”，就是经络学说的具体应用。例如：治疗胃痛，当取足阳明胃经的“足三里”穴；治疗肝病，则应刺足厥阴肝经的“期门”穴。按摩部位的选取，同样是以这一学说为依据。

中药治疗亦是通过经络这一渠道，使药达病所，以发挥其治疗作用。通过长期、反复的实践，医家们发现某一种中药对某一经脉及其所属的脏腑的病症，具有选择性的治疗作用，从而创立了“药物归经”理论。如麻黄入肺、膀胱经，故能发汗、平喘和利

Another example, thorowax root (*Radix Bupleuri*) acts on the channels of the liver and gall bladder, so as to disperse the depressed energy of the liver and gall bladder, and regulate the vital energy by alleviation of mental depression. Zhang Jiegu and Li Gao, two of the four great physicians in the Jin and Yuan dynasties, formulated a theory of "medicinal guides" according to the theory of the channels and collaterals. For instance, in treating headache, notopterygium root (*Rhizoma seu Radix Noto pterygii*) should be prescribed if it is due to *Taiyang* disturbance, or dahurian angelica root (*Radix Angeliecae Dahuricae*) should be prescribed if due to disturbance of the *Yangming*, or thorowax root (*Radix Bupleuri*) prescribed if due to disturbance of the *Shaoyang*. The above mentioned "medicinal guides" do not only work their way through the relative channel and its pertaining organ, but also direct other medicines to the right channel and organ in order to bring their therapeutic action into play.

In addition, the clinical applications of acupuncture anaesthesia, auricular needle are done under the guidance of the theory of the channels and collaterals, and will inevitably further prove and develop this theory.

尿；柴胡入肝、胆经，故可疏肝利胆，解郁理气。金元四大家中的张洁古、李杲，还根据经络学说，创立了“引经报使药”理论。如治疗头痛，属太阳经的用羌活；属阳明经的用白芷；属少阳经的用柴胡。上述“引经报使药”不仅本身进入相关经脉，而且也将别的药引入该经，以发挥其治疗作用。

此外，针刺麻醉、耳针等，也是在经络学说的指导下创立的。它们的出现将会进一步证实和发展经络学说。

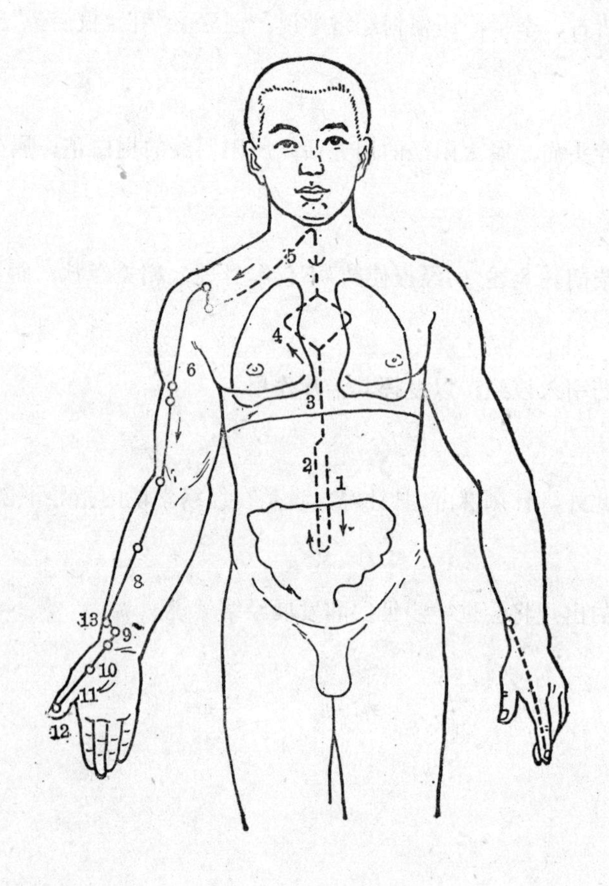

Fig. 1 The Lung Channel of Hand-*Taiyin*
图 1　手太阴肺经
Note: The unbroken line shows the channel with points
The broken line shows the internal connections of the channe without points
注：实线示本经有穴通路，虚线示本经无穴通路

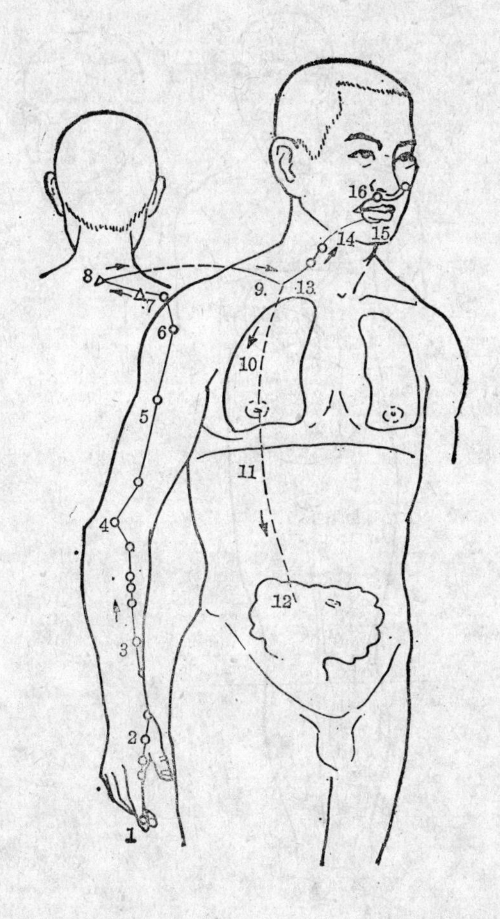

Fig. 2 The Large Intestine Channel of Hand-*Yangming*
图 2 手阳明大肠经

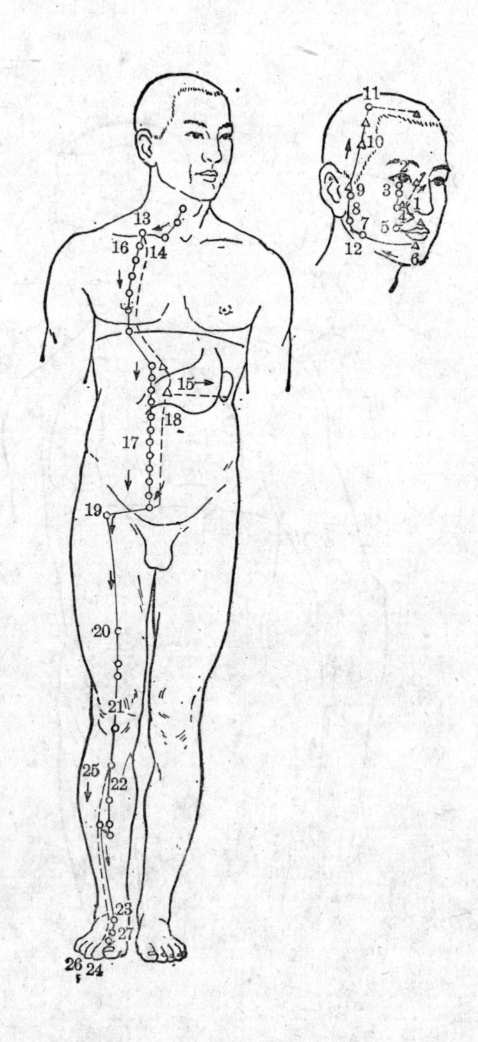

Fig. 3 The Stomach Channel of Foot-*Yangming*
图 3 足阳明胃经

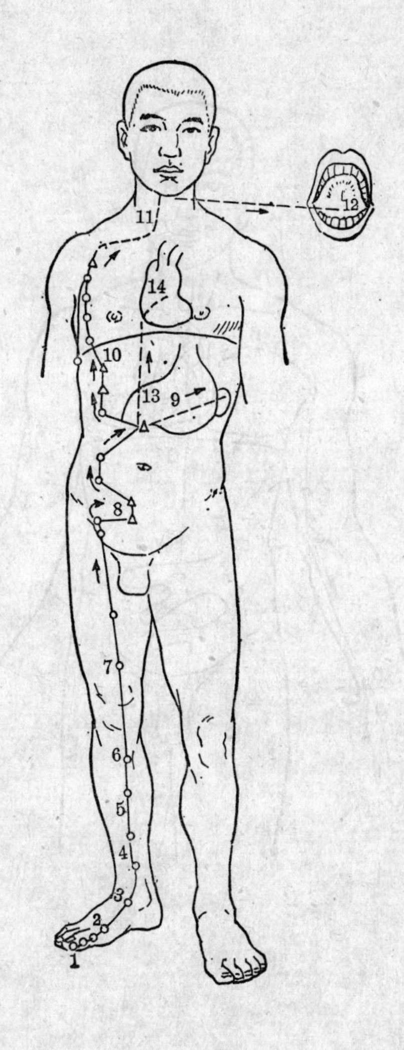

Fig. 4 The Spleen Channel of Foot-*Taiyin*
图 4 足太阴脾经

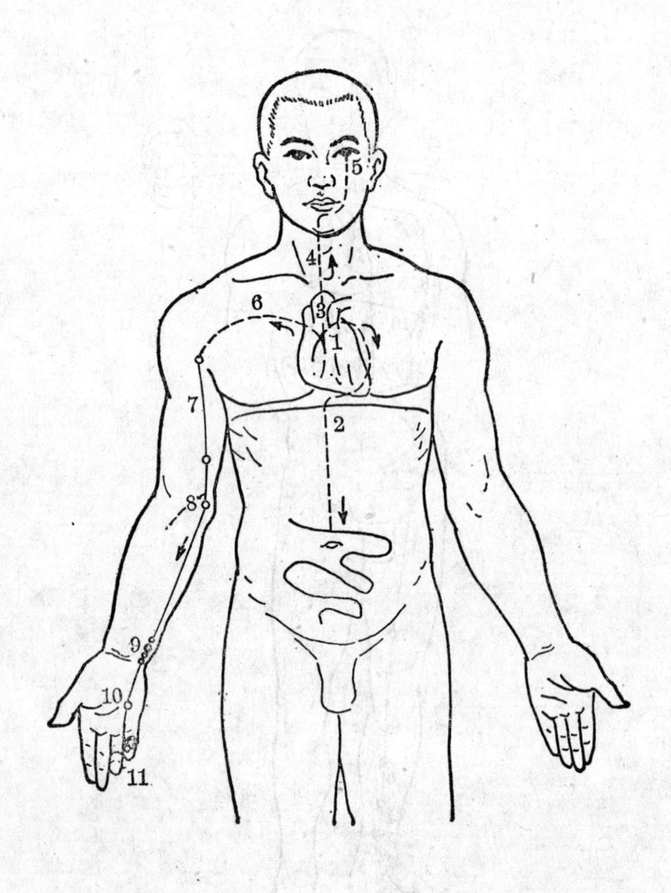

Fig. 5 The Heart Channel of Hand-*Shaoyin*
图 5 手少阴心经

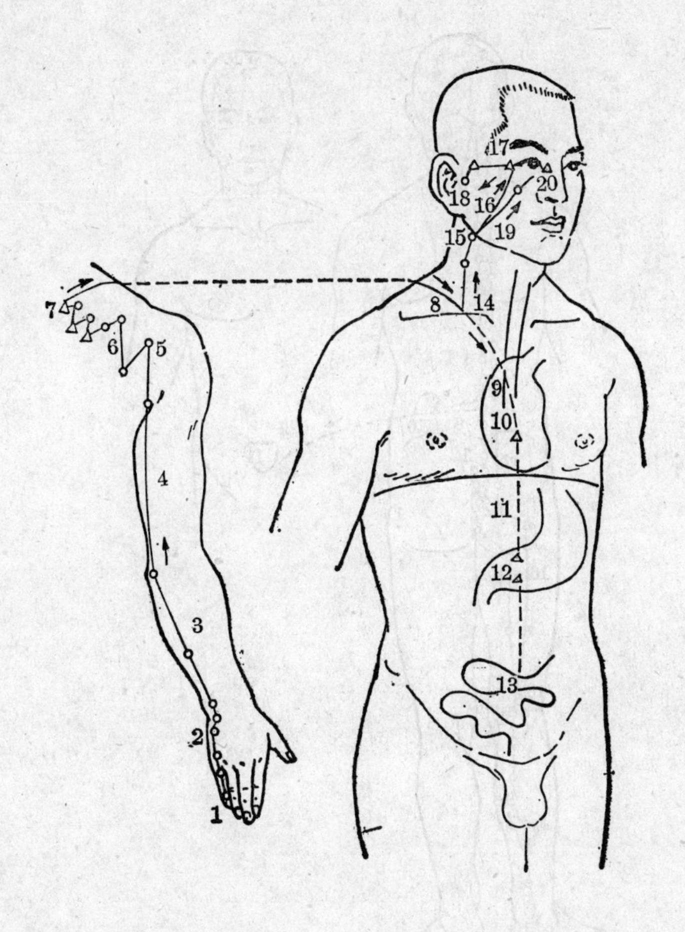

Fig. 6 The Small Intestine Channel of Hand-*Taiyang*
图 6 手太阳小肠经

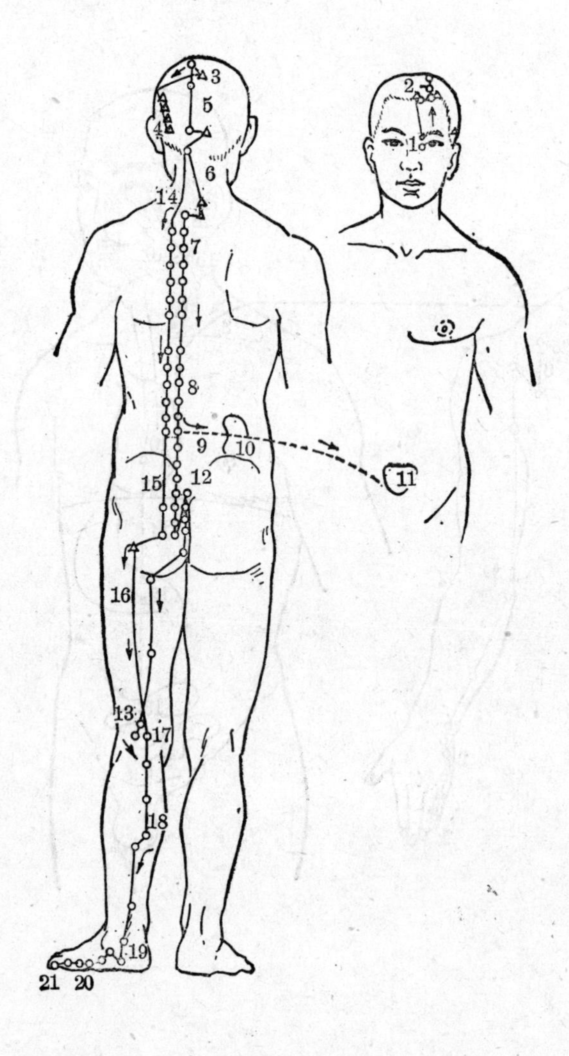

Fig. 7 The Urinary Bladder Channel of Foot-*Taiyang*
图 7 足太阳膀胱经

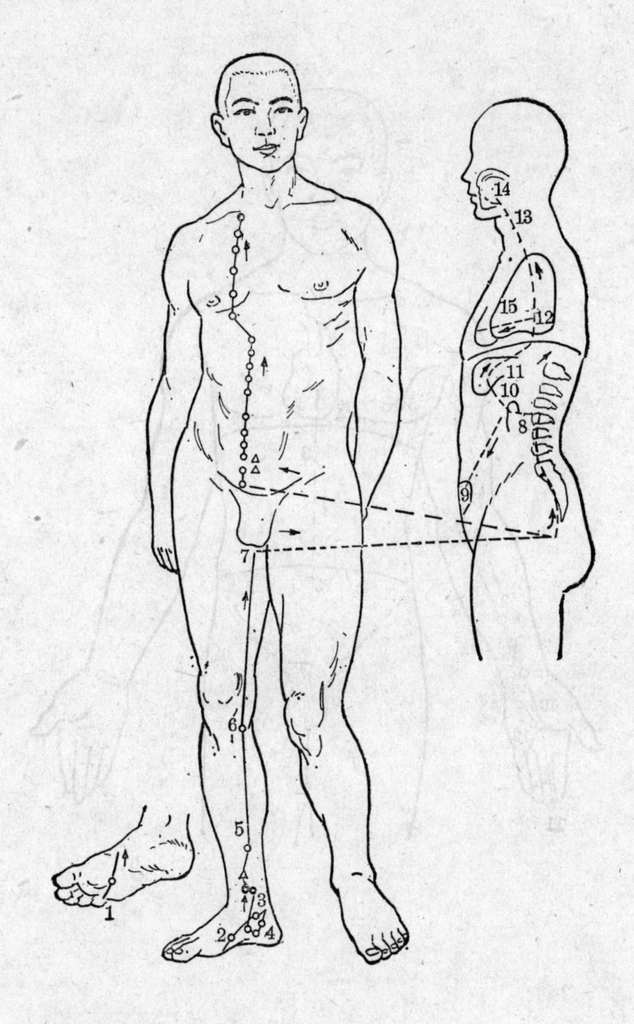

Fig. 8 The kidney Channel of Foot-*Shaoyin*
图 8 足少阴肾经

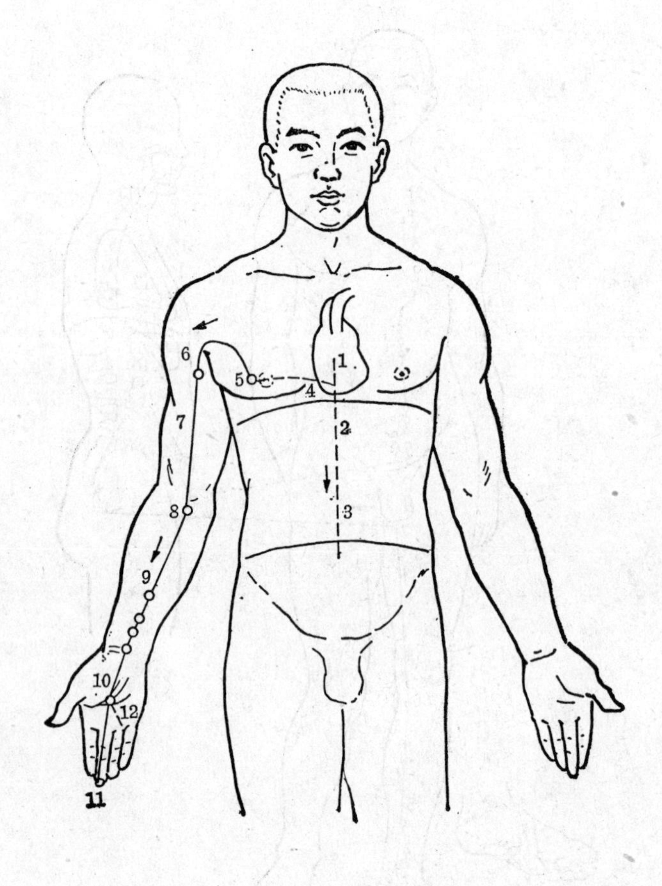

Fig. 9 The Pericardium Channel of Hand-*Jueyin*
图 9 手厥阴心包经

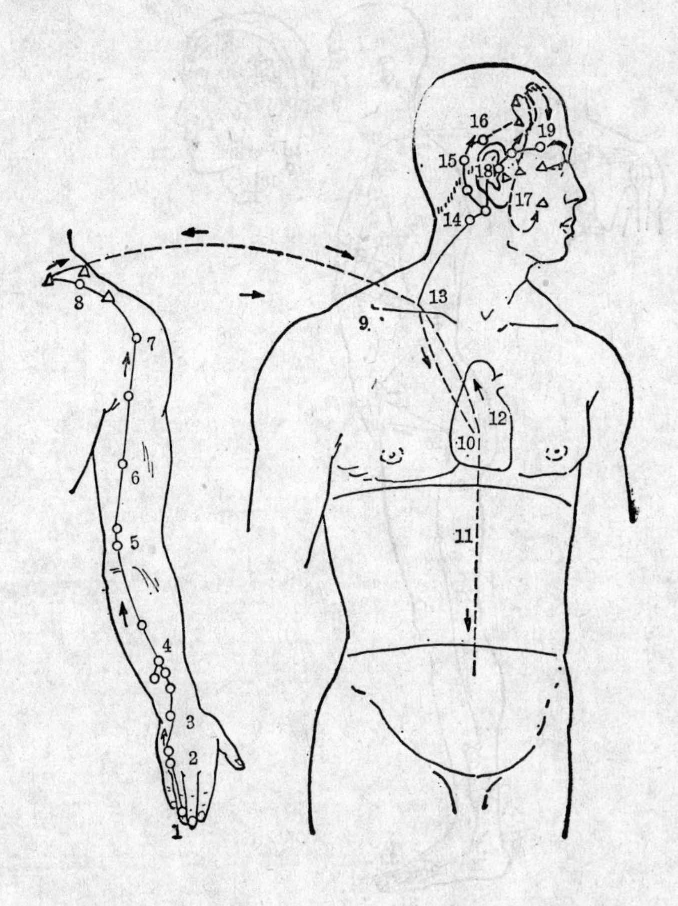

Fig. 10 The Triple Warmer Channel of Hand-*Shaoyang*
图10 手少阳三焦经

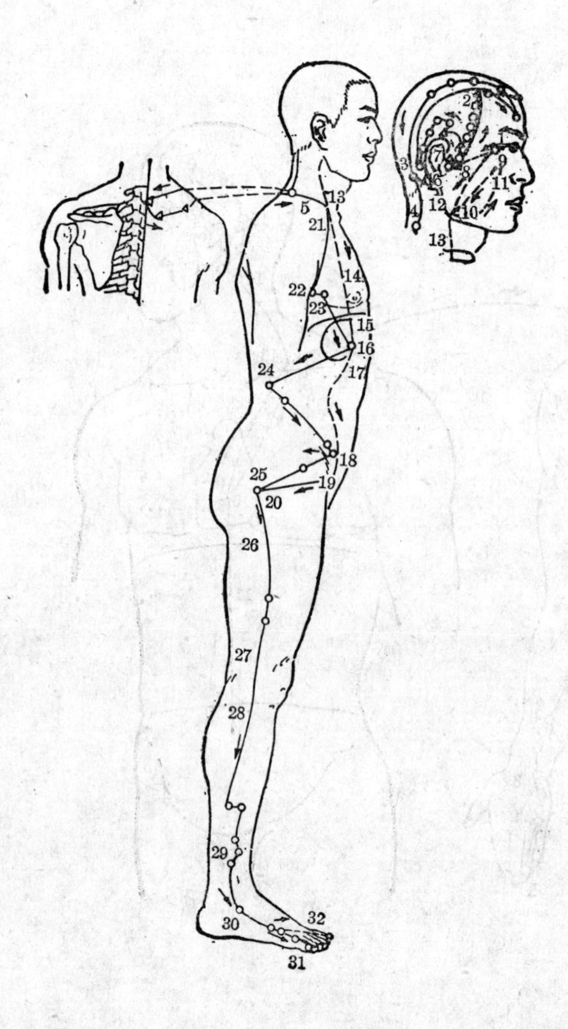

Fig. 11 The Gall Bladder Channel of Foot-*Shaoyang*
图11 足少阳胆经

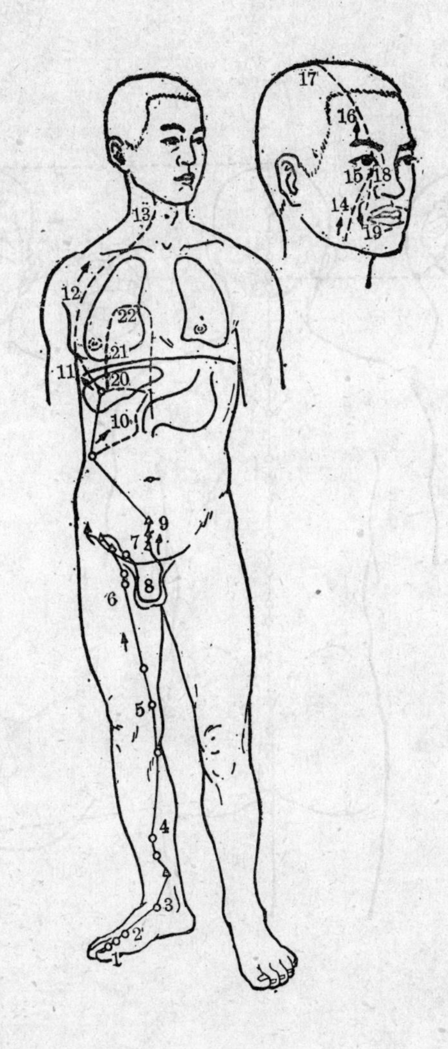

Fig. 12 The Liver Channel of Foot-*Jueyin*
图12 足厥阴肝经

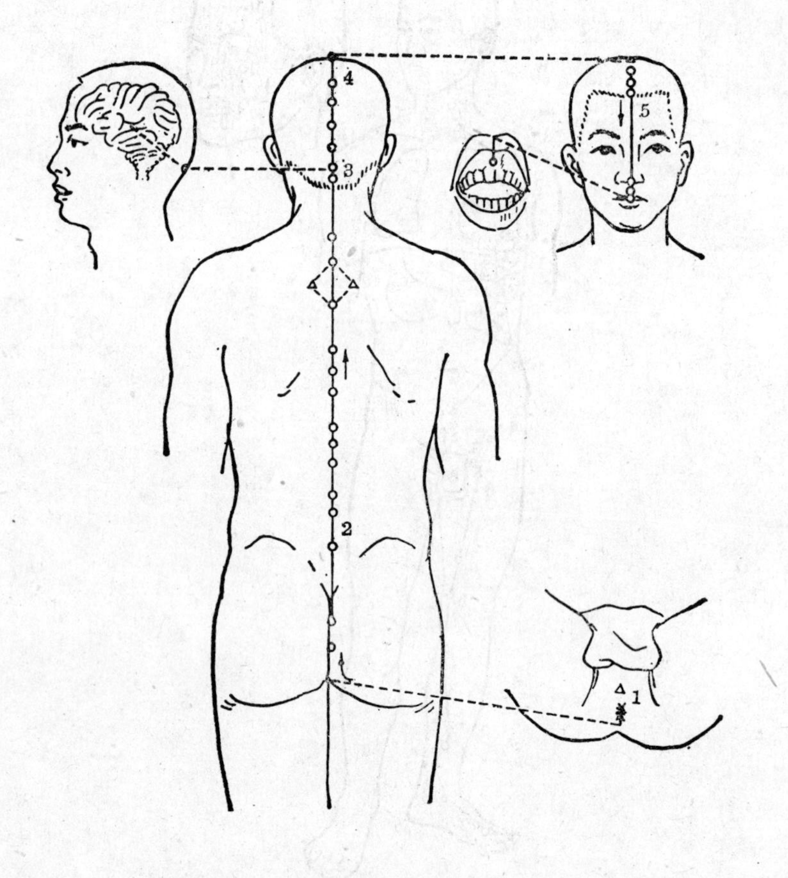

Fig. 13 The *Du* (Back Midline) Channel
图13 督脉

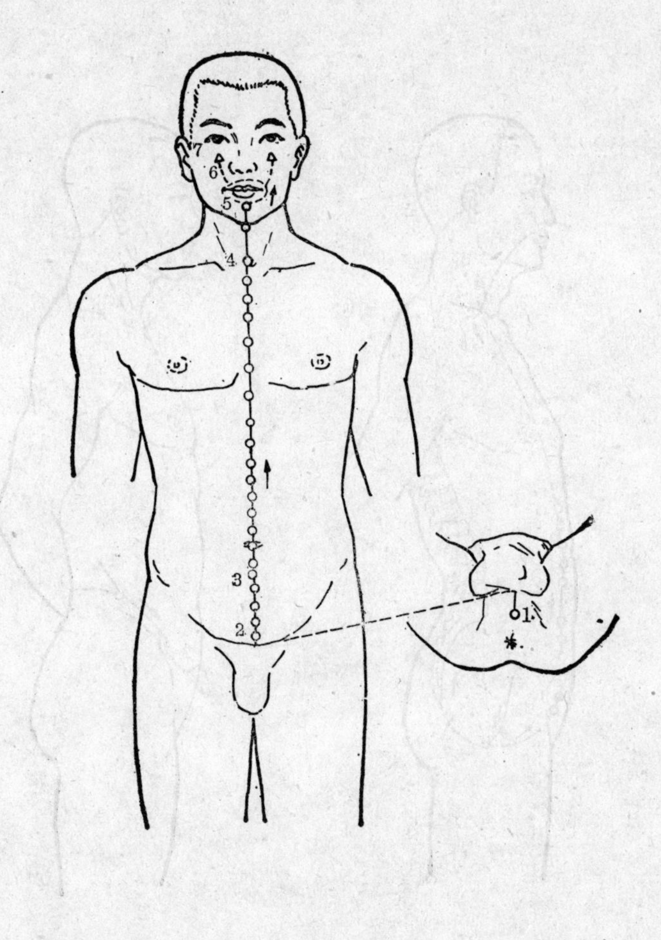

Fig. 14 The *Ren* (Front Midline) Channel
图14 任脉

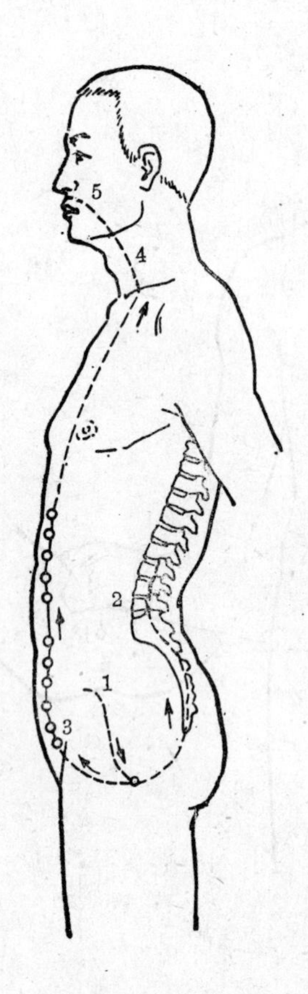

Fig. 15 The *Chong* Channel
图15 冲脉

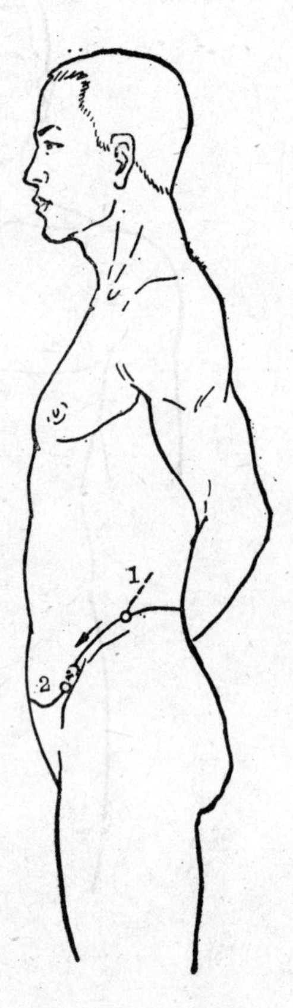

Fig. 16 The *Dai* Channel
图16 带脉

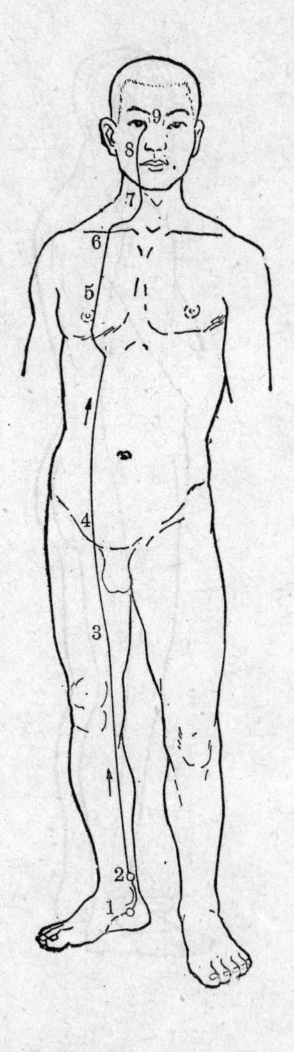

Fig. 17 The *Yinqiao* Channel
图17 阴跷脉

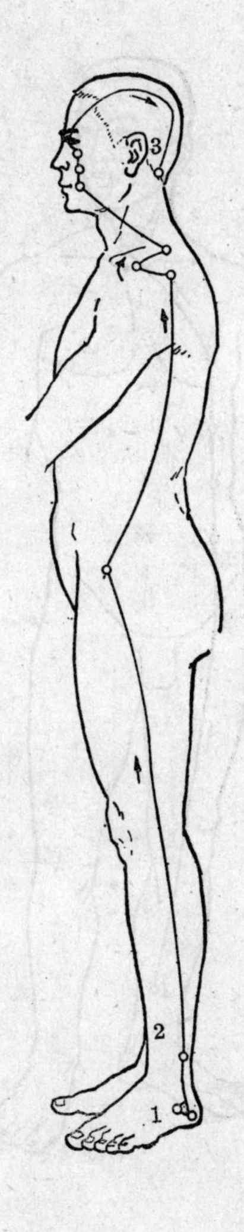

Fig. 18 The *Yangqiao* Channel
图18 阳跷脉

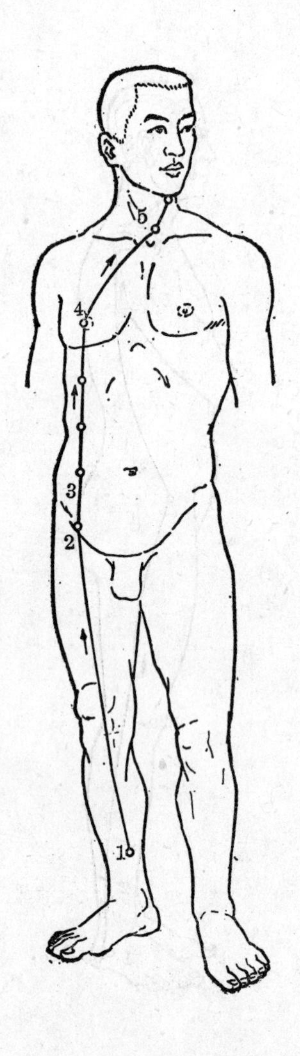

Fig. 19 The *Yinwei* Channel
图19 阴维脉

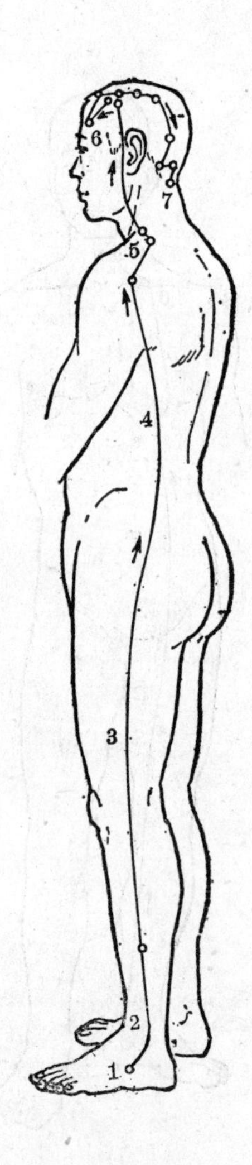

Fig. 20 The *Yangwei* Channel
图20 阳维脉

PUBLISHED ALONG WITH THE LIBRARY ARE:

- Rare Chinese Materia Medica
- Highly Efficacious Chinese Patent Medicines

《英汉对照实用中医文库》配套书

- 中国名贵药材
- 中国名优中成药

PUBLISHING HOUSE OF SHANGHAI COLLEGE OF TRADITIONAL CHINESE MEDICINE
530 Lingling Road, Shanghai, China

Chinese Massage in A Practical English – Chinese Library of TCM
Editor – in – Chief Dr. Zhangh Enqin

ISBN 7 – 81010 – 139 – 0/R. 138

Printed in Shanghai No. 3 Printing Works.

英汉对照实用中医文库
中医基础理论(上册)
主编　张恩勤
上海中医药大学出版社出版发行
(上海零陵路530号　邮政编码200032)
新华书店上海发行所经销
上海市印刷三厂印刷
开本 850×1168　1/32　印张 9.375　插页 6　字数 233千字
1990年7月第2版　　1998年8月第8次印刷
印数：19,501—22,500
ISBN 7-81010-089-0/R·88
定价：13.30元